PREFACE TO THE FOURTH EDITION

Since its first publication in 1984, the *Collins Gem Calorie Counter* has firmly established itself as one of the most successful and popular reference guides available for weight watchers.

The content of the book has been completely revised for the fourth edition. As well as data on the amount of Calories contained in a wide range of branded foods, this edition also includes figures for the amount of protein, carbohydrate, fat and dietary fibre in the products covered. Doctors and nutritionists agree that combining these ingredients in the correct proportions is essential to ensure a healthy diet.

The inclusion of this new information makes the *Collins Gem Calorie Counter* more than ever the ideal companion for the health-conscious shopper.

INTRODUCTION

For many years, doctors and successful dieters alike have acknowledged that the healthiest and most effective form of weight loss is to combine a Calorie-controlled diet with regular exercise. Now that the body's metabolism is understood more fully, the informed dieter and health-conscious eater wants to know not only the Calorie content of food but also its composition.

The body can be compared to an engine, and the 'fuel' it uses is food. About half the energy provided by food is used to keep the body functioning normally; the other half is taken up by activity such as work and recreation. Generally speaking, active people use more energy and, therefore, need to eat more to meet their energy requirements. If a person consumes more energy than he or she expends, the excess will be stored by the body as fat, and the person will put on weight. Conversely, if a person consumes less energy than he or she expends the extra energy will be taken from the body's fat stores, and the person will lose weight.

The energy provided by food and burnt up by the body is generally measured in Calories, also called kilocalories (kcal). It has been calculated that one pound of body fat is equal to 3500 Calories, so for every pound required to be lost, 3500 Calories must be burnt up or cut out of the diet over several days. On page 13 there is a table which gives the average number of Calories used in an hour taking part in certain activities. However, the rate at which the body uses up Calories varies from person to person, and depends on many factors such as a person's age, sex and general state of fitness, as well as the composition of their diet.

The food that we eat is made up of three major kinds of nutrients: *proteins, carbohydrates* and *fats*. It also provides the body with vitamins and minerals; these are called micronutrients because they are required in much smaller quantities. Nutrients all have important functions within the body.

Proteins are the building bricks of the human body. The cells of our bones, muscles, skin, nails, hair and every other tissue are made up of proteins. Many vital fluids, such as blood, enzymes and hormones, also contain proteins. There is an enormous variety of different kinds of protein, each made up of a special combination of components called amino acids.

The protein in our food is broken down into its component amino acids by the digestive system, and new proteins are synthesized by the body. The best sources of protein in the diet are meat, fish, eggs, milk and other dairy products, corn, lentils and other pulses. The protein obtained from animal sources contains more amino acids than protein from plants. Vegans, therefore, have to eat a wide variety of foods in order to ensure that their diet includes the full complement of amino acids.

Nutritionists recommend that protein represents 10% of the body's daily energy intake. This means that if a person consumes about 2400 Calories a day, 240 of those Calories should be provided by the protein in their food. One gram of protein provides about 4 Calories, so that person needs to consume about 60 grams of protein a day. Many people eat more protein than this, and there is little evidence to suggest that eating too much protein is a health risk. However, a diet low in protein is harmful, particularly to the young who are still growing.

Carbohydrates are made up of different kinds of simple sugars, such as glucose. The scientific name for the sugar that we add to our food is sucrose; one molecule or unit of sucrose is made up of two units of glucose. Carbohydrates can be divided into two different categories. The first category, which we will simply call *carbohydrates*, are known as *available carbohydrates* because the body can obtain energy from them. The second category, usually called *dietary fibres*, are known as *unavailable carbohydrates* because they are indigestible.

Available carbohydrates are important sources of energy for the body. They are broken down by the digestive system into the individual simple sugars; then they can be metabolized immediately to release energy, or they can be converted into fat and put into the body's energy stores. Starch is a form of carbohydrate, and starchy foods – such as wheat, rice, pulses and potatoes – are a good source of carbohydrates. Carbohydrates are also found in fruit and vegetables. Honey, sugar, sweets and sweetened soft drinks contain very high levels of carbohydrates, but they provide the body with virtually no other nutrients. For this reason, energy from these sources is sometimes referred to as 'empty calories'.

Although the body can obtain energy from a diet that contains no carbohydrates, they are still an important part of the diet, not least because foods rich in carbohydrates are usually good sources of micronutrients. For example, grains provide B vitamins, and fruit is an important source of vitamin C. Nutritionists recommend that 50% of the body's energy requirements are derived from carbohydrates. If a person consumes 2400 Calories a day, 1200 of those Calories should be provided by carbohydrates in their food. One gram of carbohydrate provides about 4 Calories, so that person should eat about 300 grams of carbohydrates a day.

Unavailable carbohydrates, or **dietary fibre**, cannot be broken down by the digestive system. Dietary fibre adds bulk to food and contributes to the 'full' feeling after a meal. Although it does not contain any nutrients it is an essential part of the diet and it has a number of beneficial effects, especially assisting the regular and comfortable evacuation of the bowels. Certain kinds of dietary fibre, such as oat bran, are believed to lower levels of cholesterol in the blood. Foods that contain high levels of dietary fibre are, anyway, usually good sources of other nutrients and micronutrients. They include wheat bran and bran cereals, dried fruits, nuts, pulses, and leafy green vegetables.

The average UK diet provides only about 12 grams of dietary fibre a day. Nutritionists recommend that this figure should be nearer 30 grams. If the intake of dietary fibre is increased too rapidly it may cause flatulence and diarrhoea. A very high consumption of fibre may impede the absorption of certain vital minerals.

Fats in food are the perennial enemy of the dieter. Fat has a very high energy value: 1 gram of fat provides 9 Calories; this is more than twice the calorific value of 1 gram of protein or of carbohydrate. The fat obtained from food is only broken down and used as energy when other sources of energy – carbohydrate and protein – have been exhausted. If all the fat in the diet is not converted into energy, it is simply laid down in the body's fat stores. A high intake of fats will, therefore, cause weight gain.

Vegetable oils, dripping, lard, butter, margarine, cream and nuts are all high in fat. Some meats also have a high fat content, but this can usually be reduced by trimming away the visible areas of fat before or after cooking. Fats obtained from animal sources, such as butter and cream, have been associated with an increased risk of coronary heart disease and of cancer if they are consumed in large quantities. Oils obtained from plants do not have this property, and certain vegetable and fish oils are thought to actively reduce the risk of heart disease.

Fat represents about 40% of the total energy intake of the average UK diet. This figure is much higher than it needs to be for the body's requirements. The body needs fat as an energy store and for the formation of cell membranes and the protective sheath that surrounds nerves, as well as the synthesis of certain hormones and enzymes. Most fats can be synthesized from excess carbohydrate and protein, but there are special fats called essential fatty acids which must be obtained from the diet. In order to ensure that these substances are included in the diet, fat should represent at least 2% of the body's energy intake.

However, a diet this low in fat would be unpalatable and difficult to prepare; nutritionists recommend that fat provides about 20% of the daily intake. This means that if a person consumes 2400 Calories a day, 480 of those Calories should be provided by fat in their food. Since 1 gram of fat provides 9 Calories, that person should eat about 53 grams of fat a day.

Among the tables on the following pages are those for desirable weights according to sex, height and frame. These will help to give the dieter a realistic target. Anyone considering trying to lose a lot of weight should consult their doctor, and those just keen not to overdo it should remember that the best way to lose weight – or to maintain a healthy weight – is to eat a balanced diet, to eat in moderation and to take regular exercise. Practical guidance on diet in general is given in the *Collins Gem Guide to Healthy Eating;* the *Collins Gem Guide to Food Additives* also provides essential information.

The foods in this book are listed in **bold type** in alphabetical order in the left-hand column of each page; the name of the manufacturer (of branded foods) is given in the second column. The energy value in Calories, the protein, carbohydrate, fat and dietary fibre contents per 100 gram or 100 millilitre are given in the third, fourth, fifth, sixth and seventh columns, respectively. Values for unbranded foods (listed in *bold italic type*) have been obtained from *The Composition of Foods* (5th edition, 1991) and *Vegetables, Herbs and Spices* (supplement, 1991) by permission of the Royal Society of Chemistry and the Controller of Her Majesty's Stationery Office.

The publishers are grateful to all the manufacturers who gave information on their products. The list of foods included is as up to date as it was possible to make it, but it should be remembered that new food products are frequently put on the market and existing ones withdrawn, so it has not been possible to include everything. If you cannot find a particular food here, you can still, however, obtain guideline figures by finding an equivalent product from a different manufacturer.

Weights and measures

Imperial to Metric

1 ounce (oz) = 28.35 grams (g)
1 pound (lb) = 453.60 grams (g)
1 fluid ounce (fl. oz) = 29.57 millilitres (ml)
1 pint = 0.568 litre

Metric to Imperial

100 grams (g) = 3.53 ounces (oz)
1 kilogram (kg) = 2.2 pounds (lb)
100 millilitres (ml) = 3.38 fluid ounces (fl. oz)
1 litre = 1.76 pints

Average hourly Calorie requirement by activity:

	Women	Men
Bowling	207	270
Cycling: moderate	192	256
hard	507	660
Dancing: ballroom	264	352
Domestic work	153	200
Driving	108	144
Eating	84	112
Gardening: active	276	368
Golf	144	192
Ironing	120	160
Office work: active	120	160
Rowing	600	800
Running: moderate	444	592
hard	692	900
Sewing and knitting	84	112
Sitting at rest	84	112
Skiing	461	600
Squash	461	600
Swimming: moderate	230	300
hard	480	640
Table tennis	300	400
Tennis	336	448
Typing	108	144
Walking: moderate	168	224

Desirable weight of adults: small frame

Men

Height (without shoes) ft in	m	Weight range st lb	kgs	st lb	kgs
5 1	1.55	8 0	50.8	8 8	54.4
5 2	1.58	8 3	52.2	8 12	56.3
5 3	1.60	8 6	53.5	9 0	57.2
5 4	1.63	8 9	54.9	9 3	58.5
5 5	1.65	8 12	56.3	9 7	60.3
5 6	1.68	9 2	58.1	9 11	62.1
5 7	1.70	9 6	59.9	10 1	64.0
5 8	1.73	9 10	61.7	10 5	65.8
5 9	1.75	10 0	63.5	10 10	68.0
5 10	1.78	10 4	65.3	11 0	69.9
5 11	1.80	10 8	67.1	11 4	71.7
6 0	1.83	10 12	69.0	11 8	73.5
6 1	1.85	11 2	70.8	11 13	75.8
6 2	1.88	11 6	72.6	12 3	77.6
6 3	1.91	11 10	74.4	12 7	79.4

Women

Height (without shoes) ft in	m	Weight range st lb	kgs	st lb	kgs
4 8	1.42	6 8	41.7	7 10	44.5
4 9	1.45	6 10	42.6	7 3	45.8
4 10	1.47	6 12	43.6	7 6	47.2
4 11	1.50	7 1	44.9	7 9	48.5
5 0	1.52	7 4	46.3	7 12	49.9
5 1	1.55	7 7	47.6	8 1	51.3
5 2	1.58	7 10	49.0	8 4	52.6
5 3	1.60	7 13	50.4	8 7	54.0
5 4	1.63	8 2	51.7	8 11	55.8
5 5	1.65	8 6	53.5	9 1	57.6
5 6	1.68	8 10	55.3	9 5	59.4
5 7	1.70	9 0	57.2	9 9	61.2
5 8	1.73	9 4	59.0	10 0	63.5
5 9	1.75	9 8	60.8	10 4	65.3
5 10	1.78	9 12	62.6	10 8	67.1

Desirable weight of adults: medium frame

Men

Height (without shoes) ft in m	Weight range st lb	st lb	kgs	kgs
5 1 1.55	8 6	9 3	53.5	58.5
5 2 1.58	8 9	9 7	54.9	60.3
5 3 1.60	8 12	9 10	56.3	61.7
5 4 1.63	9 1	9 13	57.6	63.1
5 5 1.65	9 4	10 3	59.0	64.9
5 6 1.68	9 8	10 7	60.8	66.8
5 7 1.70	9 12	10 12	62.6	69.0
5 8 1.73	10 2	11 2	64.4	70.8
5 9 1.75	10 6	11 6	66.2	72.6
5 10 1.78	10 10	11 11	68.0	74.8
5 11 1.80	11 0	12 2	69.9	77.1
6 0 1.83	11 4	12 7	71.7	79.4
6 1 1.85	11 8	12 12	73.5	81.7
6 2 1.88	11 13	13 3	75.8	83.9
6 3 1.91	12 4	13 8	78.0	86.2

Women

Height (without shoes) ft in m	Weight range st lb	st lb	kgs	kgs
4 8 1.42	6 12	7 9	43.6	48.5
4 9 1.45	7 0	7 12	44.5	49.9
4 10 1.47	7 3	8 1	45.8	51.3
4 11 1.50	7 6	8 4	47.2	52.6
5 0 1.52	7 9	8 7	48.5	54.0
5 1 1.55	7 12	8 10	49.9	55.3
5 2 1.58	8 1	9 0	51.3	57.2
5 3 1.60	8 4	9 4	52.6	59.0
5 4 1.63	8 8	9 9	54.4	61.2
5 5 1.65	8 12	9 13	56.3	63.1
5 6 1.68	9 2	10 3	58.1	64.9
5 7 1.70	9 6	10 7	59.9	66.7
5 8 1.73	9 10	10 11	61.7	68.5
5 9 1.75	10 0	11 1	63.5	70.3
5 10 1.78	10 4	11 5	65.3	72.1

Desirable weight of adults: large frame

Men

Height (without shoes) ft in	m	Weight range st lb	kgs	st lb	kgs
5 1	1.55	9 0	57.2	10 1	64.0
5 2	1.58	9 3	58.5	10 4	65.3
5 3	1.60	9 6	59.9	10 8	67.1
5 4	1.63	9 9	61.2	10 12	69.0
5 5	1.65	9 12	62.6	11 2	70.8
5 6	1.68	10 2	64.4	11 7	73.0
5 7	1.70	10 7	66.7	11 12	75.3
5 8	1.73	10 11	68.5	12 2	77.1
5 9	1.75	11 1	70.3	12 6	78.9
5 10	1.78	11 5	72.1	12 11	81.2
5 11	1.80	11 10	74.4	13 2	83.5
6 0	1.83	12 0	76.2	13 7	85.7
6 1	1.85	12 5	78.5	13 12	88.0
6 2	1.88	12 10	80.7	14 3	90.3
6 3	1.91	13 0	82.6	14 8	92.5

Women

Height (without shoes) ft in	m	Weight range st lb	kgs	st lb	kgs
4 8	1.42	7 6	47.2	8 7	54.0
4 9	1.45	7 8	48.1	8 10	55.3
4 10	1.47	7 11	49.4	8 13	56.7
4 11	1.50	8 0	50.8	9 2	58.1
5 0	1.52	8 3	52.2	9 5	59.4
5 1	1.55	8 6	53.5	9 8	60.8
5 2	1.58	8 9	54.9	9 12	62.6
5 3	1.60	8 13	56.7	10 2	64.4
5 4	1.63	9 3	58.5	10 6	66.2
5 5	1.65	9 7	60.3	10 10	68.0
5 6	1.68	9 11	62.1	11 0	69.9
5 7	1.70	10 1	64.0	11 4	71.7
5 8	1.73	10 5	65.8	11 9	73.9
5 9	1.75	10 9	67.6	12 0	76.2
5 10	1.78	10 13	69.4	12 5	78.5

Daily Calories for maintenance of desirable weight

Calculated for a moderately active life. If you are very active add 50 Calories; if your life is sedentary subtract 75 Calories.

Weight			Age 18–35		Age 35–55		Age 55–75	
st	lb	kgs	Men	Women	Men	Women	Men	Women
7	1	44.9		1700		1500		1300
7	12	49.9	2200	1850	1950	1650	1650	1400
8	9	54.9	2400	2000	2150	1750	1850	1550
9	2	58.1		2100		1900		1600
9	6	59.9	2550	2150	2300	1950	1950	1650
10	3	64.9	2700	2300	2400	2050	2050	1800
11	0	69.9	2900	2400	2600	2150	2200	1850
11	11	74.8	3100	2550	2800	2300	2400	1950
12	8	79.8	3250		2950		2500	
13	5	84.8	3300		3100		2600	

Abbreviations used in the Tables

g	gram
kcal	kilocalorie
ml	millilitre
N	the nutrient is present in significant quantities but there is no accurate information on the amount
n/a	not available
Tr	trace (less than 0.1g present)

A

Product	Brand	Calories kcal	Protein (g)	Carbo-hydrate (g)	Fat (g)	Dietary Fibre (g)
A1 Fruity Sauce	Sharwood	188	1.2	27.8	0.2	1.5
A La Creme Pasta Choice Dry Mix, as sold	Crosse & Blackwell	418	14.5	67.7	9.9	0.4
A La King Cook-'n-Sauce	Homepride	74.0	0.6	8.6	n/a	n/a
Abbey Crunch Biscuits	McVitie's	477	5.7	72.3	18.1	2.5
Ace, each	Lyons Maid	255	3.4	24.1	16.8	n/a
Advocaat		272	4.7	28.4	6.3	nil
Aero Chocolate Drinks, all flavours	Nestlé	97.0	4.6	12.4	3.2	0.2

All amounts given per 100g/100ml unless otherwise stated

Product	Brand	Calories kcal	Protein (g)	Carbo-hydrate (g)	Fat (g)	Dietary Fibre (g)
Aero, countline milk, peppermint, orange	Rowntree Mackintosh	527	7.7	62.0	29.3	n/a
Aero, medium orange, peppermint	Rowntree Mackintosh	527	7.7	62.0	29.3	n/a
Aero, milk chocolate	Rowntree Mackintosh	521	8.5	57.0	30.4	n/a
Aero Mini Bars	Rowntree Mackintosh	531	8.5	57.0	31.5	n/a
Aero Mousses, all flavours	Chambourcy	211	6.1	27.4	8.6	0.1
After Eight Mints	Rowntree Mackintosh	410	1.8	76.0	13.0	n/a
Alabama Chocolate Fudge Cake	McVitie's	373	4.5	61.5	12.5	0.9
Albert's Victorian Chutney	Baxters	145	0.9	37.1	0.2	2.2
Alfredo Pasta Choice Dry Mix, as sold	Crosse & Blackwell	400	16.4	60.8	10.0	0.4

All-Bran	Kellogg's	261	14.0	46.6	3.4	30.0
All Butter Shorties, each	Mr Kipling	145	1.4	16.3	8.7	n/a
All Sauce	HP	150	0.6	34.0	1.1	n/a
All Seasons Dressings (Heinz); *see flavours*						
Allinson Bread, Rolls, etc: *see flavours*						
Almond Ice Cream	Wall's Carte D'Or	120	2.5	12.0	9.0	n/a
Almond Slice	California Cake & Cookie Co.	371	12.6	50.8	17.1	n/a
each	Mr Kipling	142	1.6	20.1	4.0	n/a
Almond Slice Mix, made up per serving	Green's	164	2.5	28.0	6.0	n/a
Almond Toffee Ice Cream	Wall's Gino Ginelli Tubs	121	2.4	12.8	7.1	n/a
Almond Yorkie	Rowntree Mackintosh	528	9.5	46.9	34.9	n/a
Almonds, flaked/ground		612	21.1	6.9	55.8	12.9
Alpen	Weetabix	368	11.6	66.4	6.2	7.2

All amounts given per 100g/100ml unless otherwise stated

Product	Brand	Calories kcal	Protein (g)	Carbo-hydrate (g)	Fat (g)	Dietary Fibre (g)
no added sugar with tropical fruit	Weetabix	363	12.6	63.6	6.5	7.1
	Weetabix	369	11.4	65.0	7.0	7.5
Alphabetti Spaghetti in Tomato Sauce, reduced salt/sugar	Crosse & Blackwell	55.0	1.6	11.8	0.2	0.1
Alphabites, baked or grilled, 1oz/28g	Birds Eye	55.0	1.0	9.0	2.0	n/a
Alpine Strawberry Thick & Creamy Yogurt	Boots	113	4.9	18.0	2.9	n/a
Amber Sugar Crystals	Tate & Lyle	390	Tr	99.5	nil	nil
Ambrosia Products: see Rice, Sago, etc						
American Barbecue Beanfeast	Batchelors	307	20.7	49.6	4.2	n/a
American Broccoli Soup	Campbell's	80.0	1.3	5.3	5.9	0.2
American Brownies	California Cake & Cookie Co.	392	4.2	42.8	20.0	0.6
American Clam Chowder	Campbell's	74.0	1.8	8.0	4.1	0.4

American Ginger Ale slimline	Schweppes	21.0	n/a	5.6	n/a	n/a
	Schweppes	0.2	n/a	Tr	n/a	n/a
American Mixed Bean & Bacon Soup	Heinz	59.0	2.8	8.4	1.6	0.8
American Shoofly Pie	California Cake & Cookie Co.	440	5.5	68.0	19.1	6.5
American Style Pancake Mix, made up with milk, per serving	Green's	228	6.0	41.0	6.0	n/a
Anchovies canned in oil, drained		280	25.2	nil	19.9	nil
Anchovy Essence	Burgess	150	13.3	nil	10.4	nil
Anchovy Paste	Burgess	102	13.0	nil	5.2	nil
	Shippams	167	n/a	n/a	n/a	n/a
Angel Delight, per serving, all flavours						
made up with whole milk	Bird's	118	2.9	14.3	5.8	n/a
made up with semi-skimmed milk	Bird's	95.0	2.9	14.4	3.2	n/a
sugar free, made with						

All amounts given per 100g/100ml unless otherwise stated

Product	Brand	Calories kcal	Protein (g)	Carbo-hydrate (g)	Fat (g)	Dietary Fibre (g)
whole milk sugar free, made with semi-skimmed milk	Bird's	110	3.1	11.6	6.0	n/a
	Bird's	87.0	3.2	11.8	3.3	n/a
Angel Layer Cake	Mr Kipling	361	3.8	50.5	17.4	n/a
Animal Bar	Rowntree Mackintosh	520	8.0	58.0	30.0	n/a
Animal Biscuits	Cadbury	450	6.3	67.1	19.3	n/a
Apeel Orange Drink Mix, made up, per serving	Bird's	35.0	nil	9.0	0.1	n/a
Applause	Mars	459	6.3	65.0	21.1	2.3
Apple & Blackberry Bakewell	Mr Kipling	356	3.9	53.5	15.5	n/a
Apple & Blackberry Dumplings	McVitie's	258	3.3	35.9	11.6	0.9
Apple & Blackberry Hot Cake	McVitie's	306	3.8	41.8	14.3	1.3
Apple & Blackberry Sponge Pudding	Heinz	277	2.7	44.4	9.8	0.9

Apple & Blackberry Yogurt custard style low fat	Boots	135	4.0	19.0	5.3	n/a
	Boots	96.0	4.6	17.0	1.1	n/a
Apple & Blackcurrant Crumble	Mr Kipling	261	2.0	43.9	9.9	n/a
Apple & Blackcurrant Drink, diluted	Quosh	25.0	n/a	6.8	n/a	n/a
Apple & Blackcurrant Juice	Robinsons	19.2	Tr	n/a	Tr	n/a
Apple & Blackcurrant Pies, each individual, each	Mr Kipling	186	2.0	29.4	7.4	n/a
	Mr Kipling	426	4.4	71.4	15.6	n/a
Apple & Blackcurrant slice, each	Mr Kipling	136	1.5	20.2	6.0	n/a
Apple & Damson Yogurt, low fat	Holland & Barrett	97.0	5.4	16.9	0.8	nil
Apple & Oatbran Original Crunchy Bar	Jordans	399	9.0	50.1	20.1	5.5

All amounts given per 100g/100ml unless otherwise stated

Product	Brand	Calories kcal	Protein (g)	Carbohydrate (g)	Fat (g)	Dietary Fibre (g)
Apple & Cinnamon Cookies	Boots	482	5.1	63.0	25.0	3.4
Apple & Custard Pies, each	Mr Kipling	205	2.3	30.9	8.8	n/a
Apple & Hazelnut Real Fruit Le Yogurt, stirred, low fat	Chambourcy	102	5.3	16.4	1.7	0.1
Apple & Onion Spread	Granose	820	0.8	7.4	87.5	n/a
Apple & Raisins Harvest Chewy Bar, each	Quaker	106	1.4	17.1	3.4	0.9
Apple & Raspberry Juice Drink, diluted	Robinsons	20.4	Tr	n/a	Tr	n/a
Apple & Strawberry Juice	Copella	39.0	n/a	10.1	nil	Tr
Apple & Strawberry Juice Drink	Robinsons	22.0	Tr	n/a	Tr	n/a
Apple Bakewell	Mr Kipling	388	3.8	55.3	18.4	n/a
Apple 'C'	Libby	47.0	Tr	11.7	Tr	nil
Apple Chews, each	Trebor Bassett	13.0	Tr	3.3	0.2	n/a

Apple Chewy Bar	Boots	367	6.9	64.0	11.0	3.5
Apple Chutney		201	0.9	52.2	0.2	1.2
Apple Crumble	McVitie's	252	3.3	41.8	8.4	0.9
	Mr Kipling	242	2.0	38.6	9.9	n/a
Apple Custard Style Yogurt, low fat	Boots	91.0	4.4	17.0	1.1	n/a
Apple Drink sparkling	St Clements	43.0	nil	11.5	nil	n/a
	St Clements	43.0	n/a	n/a	n/a	n/a
	Tango	37.0	n/a	9.8	n/a	n/a
Apple Dumplings	McVitie's	258	3.5	36.7	11.2	0.9
Apple Fruit Juice	Del Monte	43.0	0.1	11.1	Tr	n/a
Apple Fruit Pie	Lyons	366	2.9	59.3	14.7	1.5
Apple Juice, unsweetened	Robinsons	38.0	0.1	9.9	0.1	Tr
Apple Juice Drink		19.6	Tr	n/a	Tr	n/a
Apple Pie dessert	McVitie's	235	2.8	35.3	9.6	0.9
popular	Lyons	349	3.0	5.1	13.6	1.5
	Lyons	344	2.7	59.4	12.3	1.5

All amounts given per 100g/100ml unless otherwise stated

Product	Brand	Calories kcal	Protein (g)	Carbo-hydrate (g)	Fat (g)	Dietary Fibre (g)
Apple Pies, each	Mr Kipling	189	2.0	30.5	7.4	n/a
individual, each	Mr Kipling	460	4.2	80.6	15.7	n/a
Apple, Raisin & Cinnamon Yogurt, low fat	Boots	91.0	4.5	17.0	1.0	n/a
Apple, Raisin & Nuts Yogurt, low fat	Boots Shapers	47.0	4.5	7.0	0.3	0.2
Apple Rice	Ambrosia	101	3.3	16.0	2.7	n/a
Apple Sauce	Colman's	86.0	0.2	n/a	Tr	n/a
	Heinz	65.0	0.2	17.2	Tr	1.7
Apple Strudel Yogurt	Alpine Ski	92.0	5.0	17.5	0.7	n/a
Apple Sultana Bran Muffin	California Cake & Cookie Co.	319	4.3	89.7	12.0	7.3
Apples, cooking						
raw, peeled		35.0	0.3	8.9	0.1	2.2
stewed with sugar		74.0	0.3	19.1	0.1	1.8
stewed without sugar		33.0	0.3	8.1	0.1	1.8

Apples, eating, average, raw		47.0	0.4	11.8	0.1	2.0
Apricot & Apple Real Fruit Le Yogurt, stirred, low fat	Chambourcy	89.0	5.0	16.9	0.6	Tr
Apricot & Coconut Ostlers	Lyons	401	5.6	61.1	16.6	9.1
Apricot & Date Bar, each	Granose	85.0	1.6	15.7	0.8	4.9
Apricot & Grapefruit Le Yogurt Actif, stirred	Chambourcy	105	4.3	14.7	3.2	0.7
Apricot & Guava Yogurt	Gold Ski	109	5.6	16.5	2.8	n/a
Apricot & Mango Yogurt	St Ivel Real	90.0	4.9	15.3	1.1	n/a
extrafruit	Ski	92.0	5.0	17.4	0.7	n/a
Greek style	St Ivel Prize	140	3.7	16.6	6.6	n/a
low calorie	St Ivel Shape	43.0	5.1	5.9	0.1	n/a
thick & creamy	Boots	113	4.9	18.0	2.9	n/a
Apricot & Nectarine Country Delight Soya Dessert	Granose	97.0	1.4	15.3	3.8	n/a
Apricot & Peach Yogurt, low fat	Boots	96.0	4.6	18.0	1.1	n/a

All amounts given per 100g/100ml unless otherwise stated

Product	Brand	Calories kcal	Protein (g)	Carbo-hydrate (g)	Fat (g)	Dietary Fibre (g)
Apricot & Starfruit Tropical Yogurt	St Ivel Shape	42.0	4.7	6.0	0.1	n/a
Apricot Chutney	Sharwood	134	0.4	33.7	0.2	0.9
Apricot Fromage Frais	St Ivel Shape	43.0	6.8	3.5	0.2	n/a
Apricot Fruit Pie	Lyons	375	3.4	63.1	13.9	2.6
Apricot Fruit Snack Bar, each	Granose	82.0	1.2	16.7	1.2	1.7
Apricot Halves in Syrup	Del Monte	73.0	0.4	18.5	0.2	n/a
	Libby	74.0	0.4	18.0	Tr	0.4
Apricot Jam	Applefords	123	0.6	23.0	Tr	n/a
	Baxters	200	Tr	53.0	nil	1.1
diabetic	Boots	165	0.2	65.0	nil	0.9
	Dietade	246	0.2	65.3	n/a	n/a
reduced sugar	Heinz Weight Watchers	134	0.4	33.0	Tr	0.7
Apricot Madeleines	Lyons	331	3.2	59.1	10.7	4.0
Apricot Rice	Ambrosia	101	3.3	16.0	2.6	n/a

Apricot Soya Yogurt	Granose	71.0	3.0	11.7	1.7	n/a
Apricot Sundae Yogurt	St Ivel Shape	47.0	4.7	7.1	0.1	n/a
Apricot Yogurt						
Greek style	Boots	142	4.4	12.0	8.8	n/a
lightly whipped	St Ivel Prize	133	4.3	14.9	6.4	n/a
Apricots, raw		31.0	0.9	7.2	0.1	1.4
canned in syrup		63.0	0.4	16.1	0.1	1.2
canned in juice		34.0	0.5	8.4	0.1	1.2
Arctic Prince Prawns	Young's	70.0	16.4	n/a	0.5	n/a
Arctic Prince Scampi	Young's	231	9.2	14.2	15.5	0.6
Arctic Roll	Birds Eye	214	3.9	39.2	5.8	n/a
Ardennes Pate	Delight	202	13.0	4.0	15.0	n/a
reduced calorie	Boots Shapers	178	17.0	3.0	11.0	n/a
Aromat	Knorr	175	12.7	26.4	2.8	0.7
Artichoke, globe, raw		18.0	2.8	2.7	0.2	N
boiled		8.0	1.2	1.2	0.1	N
Artichoke, Jerusalem, boiled		41.0	1.6	10.6	0.1	N

All amounts given per 100g/100ml unless otherwise stated

Product	Brand	Calories kcal	Protein (g)	Carbo-hydrate (g)	Fat (g)	Dietary Fibre (g)
Asparagus, raw		25.0	2.9	2.0	0.6	1.7
boiled		13.0	1.6	0.7	0.4	0.7
canned, drained		24.0	3.4	1.5	0.5	2.9
Asparagus Cuts	Green Giant	16.0	n/a	n/a	nil	n/a
Asparagus Spears						
canned	Green Giant	16.0	n/a	n/a	nil	n/a
frozen	Findus	18.0	2.6	1.1	0.4	0.8
Assorted Fruit Crumbles, each	Mr Kipling	171	2.1	28.4	6.2	n/a
Assorted Fruit Pies, each	Mr Kipling	190	2.0	30.7	7.4	n/a
Assorted Tools	Trebor Bassett	600	9.0	n/a	n/a	n/a
Aubergine, sliced, fried		302	1.2	2.8	31.9	2.9
Aurora Pasta Sauce	Dolmio	70.0	1.2	6.5	4.5	n/a
Austrian Smoked Cheese	St Ivel	315	21.0	Tr	25.0	nil
Avocado Pear, average		190	1.9	1.9	19.5	3.4

32

B

Baby Bakers	McCain	99.0	2.4	21.5	0.9	n/a
Baby Carrots, 1oz/28g	Birds Eye	6.0	1.5	33.0	Tr	n/a
Baby Cobs, frozen	Green Giant	39.0	n/a	n/a	0.5	n/a
Baby Corn Cobs	Green Giant	25.0	n/a	n/a	0.5	n/a
Baby Potatoes in Minted Butter	Ross	103	1.9	15.3	4.3	1.1
Baby Ribena Juice, undiluted						
apple	SmithKline Beecham	316	Tr	84.0	nil	nil
blackcurrant	SmithKline Beecham	316	0.1	84.0	nil	nil
orange	SmithKline					

All amounts given per 100g/100ml unless otherwise stated

Product	Brand	Calories kcal	Protein (g)	Carbo-hydrate (g)	Fat (g)	Dietary Fibre (g)
	Beecham	316	0.5	84.0	nil	nil
Baby Sweetcorn: see Sweetcorn						
Bacon, collar joint						
lean & fat, boiled		325	20.4	nil	27.0	nil
lean only, boiled		191	26.0	nil	9.7	nil
Bacon, gammon						
joint, lean & fat, boiled		269	24.7	nil	18.9	nil
joint, lean only, boiled		167	29.4	nil	5.5	nil
Bacon, rashers						
lean only, fried (average)		332	32.8	nil	22.3	nil
lean only grilled (average)		292	30.5	nil	18.9	nil
back, lean & fat, fried		465	24.9	nil	40.6	nil
middle, lean & fat, fried		477	24.1	nil	42.3	nil
middle, lean & fat, grilled		416	24.9	nil	35.1	nil
streaky, lean & fat, fried		496	23.1	nil	44.8	nil
streaky, lean & fat, grilled		422	24.5	nil	36.0	nil
Bacon Supernoodles	Batchelors	474	7.4	56.2	26.0	n/a

Bacon Wotsits, per pack	Golden Wonder	108	1.3	12.2	6.3	n/a
Baked Beans, canned in tomato sauce		84.0	5.2	15.3	0.6	6.9
	Crosse & Blackwell	75.0	5.0	12.7	0.5	6.0
	Heinz	74.0	5.0	12.7	0.3	7.3
	HP	69.0	5.0	11.0	0.5	7.3
curried with sultanas	Heinz	117	5.3	20.7	1.4	6.4
healthy balance	Crosse & Blackwell	72.0	5.0	12.0	0.4	6.0
healthy choice	HP	57.0	5.0	8.3	0.5	7.3
no added sugar	Heinz Weight Watchers	56.0	4.8	8.4	0.3	7.3
reduced sugar		73.0	5.4	12.5	0.6	7.1
with bacon	Heinz	100	7.2	15.7	0.9	5.5
with bacon burgers	HP	99.0	6.2	13.9	2.1	0.7
with beefburgers	HP	90.0	6.5	10.5	2.5	5.0
with burgerbites	Heinz	122	7.3	15.4	3.5	7.3
with low fat pork sausages	Crosse & Blackwell	91.0	6.5	10.2	2.7	5.5
with mini sausages	Heinz	120	5.3	14.6	4.5	6.5

All amounts given per 100g/100ml unless otherwise stated

Product	Brand	Calories kcal	Protein (g)	Carbohydrate (g)	Fat (g)	Dietary Fibre (g)
with pepperoni with pork sausages in tomato sauce	Heinz	109	6.4	14.5	2.8	5.6
with veg. sausage in tomato sauce	Heinz Crosse & Blackwell	110	5.2	13.0	4.1	5.2
		120	5.3	12.9	5.3	3.6
Baked Potatoes, old, with flesh & skin		136	3.9	31.7	0.2	2.7
Bakers Yeast: see Yeast						
Bakewell Slice each	Mr Kipling Peek Frean	162	1.6	22.9	7.7	n/a
		454	6.3	57.5	23.7	1.2
Bakewell Tart	McVitie's Mr Kipling	370	4.8	46.6	19.3	2.3
		414	4.2	63.8	17.5	n/a
Baking Powder		163	5.2	37.8	Tr	nil
Balmoral Shortbread	Crawfords	528	6.1	63.4	27.2	2.0
Bamboo Shoots, canned	Sharwood	11.0	1.5	0.7	0.2	1.7
		6.0	0.8	0.3	0.2	1.6

Banana & Toffee Trembler	St Ivel Fiendish Feet	71.0	2.7	15.2	0.4	n/a	n/a
Banana Blancmange	Brown & Polson	326	0.4	86.5	0.1	n/a	
Banana Cake	California Cake & Cookie Co.	328	2.9	60.1	10.0	1.28	
Banana Chips, dried	Whitworths	522	1.0	55.7	34.3	2.2	
Banana Crusha	Burgess	117	0.1	27.7	Tr	0.5	
Banana, Date & Walnut Muffin	California Cake & Cookie Co.	372	4.0	51.2	17.8	3.7	
Banana Nesquik	Nestlé	394	nil	97.3	0.5	nil	
made up with whole milk	Nestlé	168	6.8	18.9	7.8	n/a	
with semi-skimmed	Nestlé	131	6.8	18.9	3.7	n/a	
ready to drink	Nestlé	68.0	3.2	10.0	1.7	nil	
Banana Soya Milk	Granose	60.0	3.47	7.2	2.0	n/a	
Banana Yogurt	St Ivel Real	91.0	4.9	15.7	0.1	n/a	
custard style, low fat	Boots	91.0	4.5	17.0	1.0	n/a	
	Ski Classic	93.0	5.0	17.0	0.7	n/a	

All amounts given per 100g/100ml unless otherwise stated

Product	Brand	Calories kcal	Protein (g)	Carbohydrate (g)	Fat (g)	Dietary Fibre (g)
Greek style	Boots	142	4.9	13.0	8.2	n/a
Bananas		95.0	1.2	23.2	0.3	3.1
Barbecue Beans	Heinz	90.0	5.3	16.4	0.4	5.8
Barbecue Chicken Cook In The Pot Dry Mix, as sold	Crosse & Blackwell	323	11.0	50.0	8.8	2.3
Barbecue Mello 'n' Mild	Colman's	143	3.8	n/a	2.9	n/a
Barbecue Relish	Burgess	136	1.8	29.3	0.7	1.0
Barbecue Sauce	Burgess	75.0	1.8	12.2	1.8	N
	HP	118	1.7	25.8	0.2	0.9
	Homepride	140	1.0	32.0	0.8	n/a
Cook In		81.0	0.8	15.0	n/a	n/a
Barbecue Sausages Pizza	McCain Pizza Pantry	194	7.6	31.0	5.3	n/a
Barbecue Stir Fry Sauce	Uncle Ben's	127	0.6	31.3	Tr	n/a
Barbecued Beef Crisps, per pack	Golden Wonder	152	2.1	12.3	10.5	n/a

Barley Sugar, each	Trebor Bassett	23.0	n/a	6.0	n/a	n/a
diabetic	Boots	241	Tr	99.0	0.4	Tr
Basmati Rice	Uncle Ben's	142	4.0	33.0	0.3	n/a
	Whitworths	339	7.4	79.8	0.5	2.4
Bath Buns	Sunblest	296	7.3	57.1	4.3	2.2
Bath Oliver Biscuits	Fortts	412	8.4	65.5	14.8	2.7
Battenburg Cake	Lyons	373	5.1	68.2	10.7	1.3
	Mr Kipling	344	4.5	67.9	8.1	n/a
Battenburg Treats, each	Mr Kipling	156	0.8	27.1	5.6	n/a
Batter Mix						
pancake	Homepride	172	6.0	28.0	4.0	n/a
quick	Whitworths	338	9.3	77.2	1.2	3.7
Yorkshire pudding	Homepride	240	8.0	34.0	8.0	n/a
Bavarian Style Sandwich Cake Mix, per serving	Green's	255	3.0	42.0	10.0	n/a
Bavarois Chocolate Classic Dessert	Chambourcy	189	3.8	25.2	8.0	0.3

All amounts given per 100g/100ml unless otherwise stated

Product	Brand	Calories kcal	Protein (g)	Carbo-hydrate (g)	Fat (g)	Dietary Fibre (g)
Bavarois Raspberry Classic Dessert	Chamboury	162	2.6	25.5	5.5	0.5
Bean & Mushroom Stew	Granose	78.0	3.0	14.0	1.0	0.2
Bean Salad & Chicken, per pack	Boots	208	n/a	n/a	n/a	n/a
Beanfeast (Batchelors): see flavours						
Beans: see types						
Beans, refried	Old El Paso	94.0	n/a	n/a	n/a	n/a
Beans & Hot Dogs in Smokey Bacon Sauce	Heinz	123	4.8	13.6	5.9	4.8
Beansprouts, mung, raw						
boiled		31.0	2.9	4.0	0.5	5.6
canned		25.0	2.5	2.8	0.5	1.3
stir fried in oil		10.0	1.6	0.8	0.1	0.7
		25.0	1.9	2.5	6.1	0.9
Beansprouts Stir Fry	Uncle Ben's	54.0	0.6	11.8	0.5	n/a
Beef						
brisket lean & fat, boiled		326	27.6	nil	23.9	nil

forerib, roast		349	22.4	nil	28.8	nil
mince, stewed		229	23.1	nil	15.2	nil
rump steak, lean & fat, fried		246	28.6	nil	14.6	nil
rump steak, lean & fat, grilled		218	27.3	nil	12.1	nil
rump steak, lean only, fried		190	30.8	nil	7.4	nil
rump steak, lean only, grilled		168	28.6	nil	6.0	nil
silverside, lean & fat, boiled		242	28.6	nil	14.2	nil
silverside, lean only, boiled		173	32.3	nil	4.9	nil
sirloin, lean & fat, roast		284	23.6	nil	21.1	nil
sirloin, lean only, roast		192	27.6	nil	9.1	nil
stewing steak, lean & fat, stewed		223	30.9	nil	11.0	nil
topside, lean & fat, roast		214	26.6	nil	12.0	nil
topside, lean only, roast		156	29.2	nil	4.4	nil
Beef & Chilli Bean Soup	Campbell's	65.0	4.3	10.7	0.9	3.0
Beef & Kidney	Tyne Brand	116	10.9	2.0	7.2	n/a
Beef & Kidney Pie	Tyne Brand	159	7.0	11.2	9.9	n/a
Beef & Mushroom Pie	Tyne Brand	152	5.9	10.7	9.8	n/a
Beef & Onion, minced	Tyne Brand	116	9.0	7.0	6.0	n/a

All amounts given per 100g/100ml unless otherwise stated

Product	Brand	Calories kcal	Protein (g)	Carbohydrate (g)	Fat (g)	Dietary Fibre (g)
Beef & Vegetable Soup	Campbell's Main Course	38.0	2.6	6.3	0.2	1.0
	Heinz Big Soups	37.0	2.2	6.4	0.3	0.8
Beef Bolognese Cook In The Pot Microwave Mix, as sold	Crosse & Blackwell	316	12.1	53.3	6.0	3.8
Beef Bourguignon Casserole Mix	Colman's	314	5.4	n/a	1.7	n/a
Beef Broth	Heinz Big Soups	31.0	1.6	5.4	0.3	0.7
	Heinz Farmhouse	40.0	1.6	7.1	0.6	0.5
Beef Cannelloni	Findus Dinner Supreme	140	6.6	12.7	7.0	0.7
Beef Cantonese, per pack	Birds Eye Healthy Options	240	25.0	25.0	5.0	n/a
Beef Casserole	Batchelors Microchef Meal	85.0	7.1	7.8	3.0	n/a

	Brand						
canned	Tyne Brand	87.0	5.9	5.9	5.9	4.6	n/a
Beef Casserole with Potato Microchef Snack	Batchelors	60.0	3.8	8.2	1.3		n/a
Beef Chow Mein Instant Pot Meal	Boots Shapers	326	15.0	63.0	3.3		n/a
Beef Consommé	Baxters	12.0	2.4	0.7	Tr		nil
Beef Cubes	Knorr	334	10.8	29.5	20.0		0.5
Beef Curry							
canned	Vesta	107	3.5	18.8	2.5		n/a
	Campbell's	95.0	5.8	9.6	3.7		1.6
	Fray Bentos	109	13.5	5.9	3.7		n/a
	Tyne Brand	93.0	5.0	9.2	4.2		n/a
Favourite Recipe, per pack	Birds Eye MenuMaster	205	18.0	17.0	7.5		n/a
Microchef Meal	Batchelors	144	6.9	18.4	4.8		n/a
Beef Curry with Rice, per pack	Birds Eye MenuMaster	395	25.0	67.0	5.0		n/a
per pack	Heinz	90.0	4.3	12.9	2.4		0.9
per pack	Lunchbowl Tyne Brand	411	18.0	66.6	8.5		n/a

All amounts given per 100g/100ml unless otherwise stated

Product	Brand	Calories kcal	Protein (g)	Carbo-hydrate (g)	Fat (g)	Dietary Fibre (g)
Microchef Snack	Batchelors	199	3.5	12.2	3.5	n/a
Beef Dripping		891	Tr	Tr	99.0	nil
Beef Essence	Sharwood	25.0	6.2	0.2	n/a	n/a
Beef Goulash	Campbell's	79.0	7.0	8.5	2.1	0.5
Beef Goulash Casserole Mix	Colman's	313	6.7	n/a	3.9	n/a
Beef Goulash Cook In The Pot Dry Mix, as sold	Crosse & Blackwell	332	8.6	51.4	10.2	4.7
Beef Goulash Microchef Snack	Batchelors	58.0	3.9	8.7	1.1	n/a
Beef Goulash with Noodles	Heinz Lunchbowl	66.0	4.2	7.9	2.0	0.5
Beef Grillsteaks, grilled baked or fried, each	Birds Eye Steakhouse	165	13.0	1.0	12.0	n/a
Beef Hungarian with Vegetables & Rice	Heinz Weight Watchers	78.0	5.9	10.4	1.4	1.1
Beef in Beer Casserole						

Recipe Sauce	Knorr	44.0	0.7	10.5	0.2	n/a
Beef in Stout with Herb Dumplings, per pack	Birds Eye MenuMaster	215	19.0	18.0	8.0	n/a
Beef Julienne	Findus Lean Cuisine	100	7.3	13.2	1.9	0.7
Beef Lasagne	Boots Shapers	113	8.6	9.0	5.0	1.6
	Heinz Weight Watchers	94.0	6.1	12.0	2.4	0.5
Beef Madras Curry	Findus Dinner Supreme	152	7.0	21.5	4.9	1.0
	Vesta	105	3.6	19.4	2.0	n/a
Beef Oriental with Special Egg Rice	Heinz	86.0	4.5	12.5	2.0	0.5
Beef Paste	Shippams	201	n/a	n/a	n/a	n/a
Beef Risotto	Vesta	152	5.5	22.9	4.9	n/a
Beef Satay Stir Fry Cook In The Pot Dry Mix, as sold	Crosse & Blackwell	416	13.0	46.3	19.9	2.3

All amounts given per 100g/100ml unless otherwise stated

Product	Brand	Calories kcal	Protein (g)	Carbo-hydrate (g)	Fat (g)	Dietary Fibre (g)
Beef Sausages: see Sausages, beef						
Beef Savoury Rice	Batchelors	329	6.9	75.0	2.2	n/a
Beef Soup	Heinz	38.0	2.0	4.4	1.4	0.1
Beef Stew canned	Campbell's	120	9.7	4.6	7.2	0.7
	Tyne Brand	70.0	5.6	8.5	1.8	1.1
		75.0	5.0	7.2	3.2	n/a
Beef Stew & Dumplings, per pack	Birds Eye Trad. Recipe	350	20.0	33.0	16.0	n/a
	Tyne Brand	456	19.4	46.2	22.8	n/a
Beef Stock Powder	Knorr	196	9.7	29.4	5.3	0.2
Beef Stroganoff Casserole Mix	Colman's	317	12.0	n/a	3.0	n/a
Beef Stroganoff Cook In The Pot Dry Mix, as sold	Crosse & Blackwell	348	13.3	47.7	11.5	2.8
Beef Supernoodles	Batchelors	474	7.4	56.2	26.0	n/a
Beef Topsteak	Ross	357	15.0	nil	30.8	nil

Beef Wotsits, per pack	Golden Wonder	116	1.2	13.4	6.7	n/a
Beefburgers, fried						
economy						
100%, each	Ross	264	20.4	7.0	17.3	1.4
	Birds Eye	257	16.4	7.7	18.0	0.3
	Steakhouse	120	9.0	3.5	9.0	n/a
	Ross	335	17.5	nil	29.1	nil
lean						
low fat, each	Findus	173	16.1	2.4	11.0	0.2
	Birds Eye	85.0	9.0	2.0	4.5	n/a
original, each	Steakhouse	120	9.0	1.5	8.5	n/a
	Birds Eye					
quarterpounders, each	Steakhouse	235	17.0	3.5	17.0	n/a
	Birds Eye	294	13.9	3.4	25.0	0.3
real	Findus					
Beefeater Fast Fry Chips	McCain	101	2.4	17.4	2.4	1.5
Beer						
bitter, canned		32.0	0.3	2.3	Tr	nil
bitter, draught		32.0	0.3	2.3	Tr	nil
bitter, keg		31.0	0.3	2.3	Tr	nil

All amounts given per 100g/100ml unless otherwise stated

Product	Brand	Calories kcal	Protein (g)	Carbohydrate (g)	Fat (g)	Dietary Fibre (g)
mild, draught		25.0	0.2	1.6	Tr	nil
Beer Shandy	Corona	25.0	n/a	5.3	n/a	n/a
Beetroot, raw		36.0	1.7	7.6	0.1	2.8
boiled		46.0	2.3	9.5	0.1	2.3
pickled		28.0	1.2	5.6	0.2	2.5
pickled, all varieties	Baxters	35.0	1.8	6.8	Tr	2.5
Beetroot in Redcurrant Jelly	Baxters	167	0.7	43.9	Tr	0.9
Bemax crunchy wheatgerm	SmithKline Beecham	310	12.0	60.0	4.0	14.5
natural wheatgerm	SmithKline Beecham	300	24.0	35.5	7.8	10.0
Bengal Hot Chutney	Sharwood	230	0.5	59.8	0.4	1.1
Best Burger	Ross	285	12.4	3.4	24.7	0.1
Best English Mints	Cravens	375	nil	96.5	nil	nil
Biarritz	Cadbury	495	4.5	59.8	27.9	n/a

Big Beans in Tomato Sauce	HP	69.0	5.0	11.0	0.5	7.3
Big Mac, each	McDonald's	446	28.1	46.2	17.7	3.5
Big Soups (Heinz): see flavours						
Big Squeeze						
lemon	Lyons Maid	81.0	1.0	16.9	1.4	n/a
orange	Lyons Maid	82.0	1.0	17.2	1.4	n/a
Bigga Peas, canned	Batchelors	80.0	6.5	13.4	0.4	n/a
Biryani Curry Sauce Mix, as sold	Sharwood	230	16.4	24.7	7.4	3.1
Biscuit Base, made up	Whitworths	631	2.3	24.4	58.8	0.8
Biscuits						
chocolate, full coated		524	5.7	67.4	27.6	2.9
digestive, chocolate		493	6.8	66.5	24.1	3.1
digestive, plain		471	6.3	68.6	20.9	4.6
sandwich		513	5.0	69.2	25.9	1.1
semi-sweet		457	6.7	74.8	16.6	2.1
short-sweet		469	6.2	62.2	23.4	1.5

All amounts given per 100g/100ml unless otherwise stated

Product	Brand	Calories kcal	Protein (g)	Carbo-hydrate (g)	Fat (g)	Dietary Fibre (g)
Bisto						
original	RHM Foods	257	1.7	59.8	0.2	n/a
cheese sauce granules	RHM Foods	596	6.4	38.6	45.7	0.6
chicken gravy granules	RHM Foods	497	4.1	38.3	35.7	n/a
fuller flavour gravy granules	RHM Foods	326	7.3	63.5	3.8	1.0
onion gravy granules	RHM Foods	484	4.0	41.1	33.0	2.2
parsley gravy granules	RHM Foods	588	3.5	43.4	43.9	0.7
rich gravy granules	RHM Foods	485	3.8	37.1	35.1	0.4
Bistro Break (HP): see flavours						
Bitter: see Beer						
Bitter Lemon, sparkling	Schweppes	32.9	n/a	8.7	n/a	n/a
slimline	Schweppes	0.4	n/a	Tr	n/a	n/a
Black Bean Stir Fry Sauce	Sharwood	90.0	0.3	19.9	1.3	1.2
Black Cherries in Syrup	Libby	73.0	n/a	n/a	Tr	n/a
Black Cherry Cheesecake	Chambourcy	254	6.0	35.0	10.0	2.1
Black Cherry Cheesecake Mix, per serving	Homepride Classic	258	3.0	30.0	13.0	n/a

Black Cherry Crusha	Burgess	149	nil	36.2	nil	nil
Black Cherry Delight Dairy Ice Cream	Lyons Maid Napoli	101	1.6	17.5	0.2	n/a
Black Cherry Soya Ice Cream	Granose	96.0	1.2	14.4	3.4	n/a
Black Cherry Yogurt	St Ivel Real	90.0	4.9	15.4	1.1	n/a
	Gold Ski	111	5.3	17.2	2.8	n/a
	Ski	132	3.8	27.7	1.4	n/a
frozen	St Ivel Prize	137	4.3	15.9	6.4	n/a
lightly whipped	St Ivel Prize	63.0	3.5	12.8	0.1	n/a
long life	Boots	96.0	4.6	18.0	1.1	n/a
low calorie	St Ivel Shape	42.0	4.7	6.0	0.1	n/a
Black Forest Cream Cake	McVitie's	271	3.3	38.1	12.3	1.4
Black Forest Fromage Frais	St Ivel Shape	56.0	6.9	6.5	0.3	n/a
Black Forest Gateau	McVitie's	302	2.7	33.8	17.5	0.4
individual	St Ivel	199	3.5	21.1	11.3	n/a
Black Forest Gateau Classic Dessert	Chambourcy	207	3.3	26.7	9.7	0.4

All amounts given per 100g/100ml unless otherwise stated

Product	Brand	Calories kcal	Protein (g)	Carbo-hydrate (g)	Fat (g)	Dietary Fibre (g)
Black Forest Sundae Yogurt	St Ivel Shape	46.0	4.9	6.2	0.2	n/a
Black Jack Chews, each	Trebor Bassett	15.0	0.1	3.3	0.2	n/a
Black Magic Assortment	Rowntree Mackintosh	457	3.7	64.0	22.5	n/a
Black Magic Chocolate Bar	Rowntree Mackintosh	490	4.5	54.7	29.7	n/a
Black Pudding, fried		305	12.9	15.0	21.9	0.5
Black Treacle	Lyle's	257	1.0	64.0	nil	nil
Blackberry & Apple Crunchy Dessert Mix, per serving	Green's	258	2.0	46.0	8.0	n/a
Blackberry & Blackcurrant Le Yogurt Actif, stirred	Chambourcy	112	4.3	16.5	3.1	0.7
Blackberry & Custard Pies, each	Mr Kipling	215	2.5	32.1	9.4	n/a
Blackberry Carob Coated Fruit Snack Bar, each	Granose	168	3.2	30.6	3.7	2.3

Blackberries, raw		25.0	0.9	5.1	0.2	6.6
stewed with sugar		56.0	0.7	13.8	0.2	5.2
stewed without sugar		21.0	0.8	4.4	0.2	5.6
Blackcurrant & Apple Drink	Boots Shapers	0.2	Tr	nil	nil	nil
Blackcurrant & Apple Fruit Pie	Lyons	376	3.0	60.4	15.2	1.9
Blackcurrant & Apple Juice	Copella	50.0	n/a	12.5	nil	Tr
Blackcurrant & Apple Soya Yogurt	Granose	68.0	3.0	10.8	1.7	n/a
Blackcurrant & Liquorice	Cravens	385	1.0	89.2	4.1	nil
Blackcurrant & Raspberry Fromage Frais Split	Ski Gold	141	5.5	19.3	5.2	n/a
Blackcurrant & Raspberry Trembler	St Ivel Fiendish Feet	76.0	2.7	16.3	0.4	n/a
Blackcurrant 'C'	Libby	54.0	Tr	13.5	Tr	nil
Blackcurrant Cheesecake	Eden Vale	261	2.8	38.8	11.6	n/a
	McVities	390	4.9	31.9	22.7	0.4

All amounts given per 100g/100ml unless otherwise stated

Product	Brand	Calories kcal	Protein (g)	Carbo-hydrate (g)	Fat (g)	Dietary Fibre (g)
party	McVities	321	4.4	33.8	18.8	0.4
Blackcurrant Cheesecake Mix, made up per serving	Lyons Tetley Homepride Classic	247	4.1	29.6	12.0	n/a
		261	3.5	32.0	13.5	n/a
Blackcurrant Cordial, diluted	Britvic	21.0	n/a	5.5	n/a	n/a
Blackcurrant Creme Sundae Yogurt	St Ivel Shape	42.0	4.7	5.6	0.1	n/a
Blackcurrant Devonshire Cheesecake	St Ivel	250	6.3	26.5	14.0	n/a
Blackcurrant Drink	Boots Shapers	14.0	0.1	3.6	nil	nil
Blackcurrant Fool Mix, made up	Lyons Tetley	150	3.6	19.9	5.9	n/a
Blackcurrant Fruit Pastilles	Rowntree Mackintosh	329	4.0	83.3	nil	n/a
Blackcurrant Jam	Applefords	109	0.2	19.5	Tr	n/a

diabetic	Baxters	3.1	Tr	53.0	Tr	200
reduced sugar	Boots	1.7	nil	64.0	0.3	161
	Heinz Weight Watchers	3.0	Tr	33.0	0.4	125
Blackcurrant Juice Drink undiluted	Ribena	n/a	n/a	15.6	Tr	59.0
	Baby Ribena	n/a	n/a	84.0	Tr	316
	Ribena	n/a	n/a	76.0	Tr	285
Blackcurrant Meringue Pie Mix, per serving	Homepride Classic	n/a	5.5	27.5	2.5	171
Blackcurrant Monster Mousse	St Ivel Fiendish Feet	n/a	1.5	11.2	2.2	64.0
Blackcurrant Vitamin C Drink, undiluted	C-Vit	n/a	n/a	39.5	Tr	148
Blackcurrant Yogurt, bio, stirred	Ski	n/a	3.0	16.9	5.8	114
Blackcurrants, raw		7.8	Tr	6.6	0.9	28.0
stewed with sugar		6.1	Tr	15.0	0.7	58.0
canned in juice		4.2	Tr	7.6	0.8	31.0

All amounts given per 100g/100ml unless otherwise stated

Product	Brand	Calories kcal	Protein (g)	Carbohydrate (g)	Fat (g)	Dietary Fibre (g)
canned in syrup		72.0	0.7	18.4	Tr	3.6
Blackeye Beans, boiled		116	8.8	19.9	0.7	3.5
Bloater Paste	Shippams	171	n/a	n/a	n/a	n/a
Blue Band Margarine	Van Den Berghs	740	0.4	0.1	82.0	n/a
Blue Cheese Dressing	Kraft	482	2.0	9.0	49.0	n/a
Blue Fjord North Atlantic Peeled Prawns	Young's	70.0	16.4	nil	0.5	n/a
Blue Riband	Rowntree	530	6.0	64.0	29.5	n/a
mini	Mackintosh	521	6.3	64.8	28.1	n/a
Blue Ribbon Vanilla Ice Cream	Wall's	85.0	1.5	11.0	4.0	n/a
cream of Cornish	Wall's	90.0	2.0	12.0	4.5	n/a
cream of Cornish, low fat	Wall's	80.0	2.0	12.0	3.0	n/a
Blue Ribbon Vanilla Ice Cream Bar, each	Wall's	85.0	1.5	11.0	4.0	n/a
Blue Stilton Cheese: *see Stilton*						

Blueberry & Loganberry Fruit on Bottom Yogurt	Ski	107	5.4	16.0	2.8	n/a
Blueberry Muffin	California Cake & Cookie Co.	326	5.6	42.6	15.7	1.8
Boasters	McVitie's	547	6.3	54.8	33.1	1.8
Bodyline Cottage Cheese						
natural	Eden Vale	83.0	13.0	3.6	1.9	n/a
onion & chive	Eden Vale	81.0	12.7	3.6	1.9	n/a
pineapple	Eden Vale	82.0	11.1	6.1	1.6	n/a
Boeuf Bourguignon	Baxters	98.0	11.4	3.2	4.5	0.4
Boiled Sweets		327	Tr	87.3	Tr	nil
Bologna	Granose	167	20.1	11.7	4.7	1.5
Bolognese, canned	Fray Bentos	98.0	10.4	4.7	4.3	n/a
Bolognese Beanfeast	Batchelors	333	26.9	49.0	4.6	n/a
Bolognese Casserole Recipe Sauce	Knorr	62.0	1.7	7.4	3.0	n/a
Bolognese Sauce, cooked		145	8.0	3.7	11.1	1.1

All amounts given per 100g/100ml unless otherwise stated

Product	Brand	Calories kcal	Protein (g)	Carbo-hydrate (g)	Fat (g)	Dietary Fibre (g)
	Buitoni	60.0	3.3	9.1	0.9	0.3
	Dolmio	95.0	5.8	7.0	5.0	n/a
with mushrooms	Buitoni	60.0	3.8	9.5	0.9	0.6
with peppers (& meat)	Buitoni	65.0	3.8	9.7	1.0	0.6
with peppers (no meat)	Buitoni	91.0	1.8	18.7	0.8	0.8
Bombay Mix		5.3	18.8	35.1	32.9	6.2
Bombay Spiced Poppadums	Sharwood	301	22.7	61.9	3.6	14.5
Bombay Vegetable Biryani Microwave Meal	Sharwood	141	3.6	17.2	6.2	1.2
Bon Bons, all flavours, each	Trebor Bassett	27.0	1.0	5.9	0.4	n/a
Boost, per bar						
biscuit	Cadbury	280	4.0	34.0	15.1	n/a
coconut	Cadbury	270	4.5	27.2	16.9	n/a
peanut	Cadbury	270	5.7	27.5	15.7	n/a
Boots Shapers Products: see flavours						
Borlotti Beans	Napolina	70.0	4.9	12.8	0.3	5.5

Bounty, milk chocolate	Mars	471	4.6	56.4	26.8	3.8
plain chocolate	Mars	467	3.2	57.4	26.5	3.8
Bourbon Biscuits	Peek Frean	464	4.8	66.5	21.7	1.5
Bourbon Creams	Crawfords	485	4.7	70.2	20.4	1.5
Bourguignon Cook-In-Sauce	Homepride	46.0	0.7	10.1	n/a	n/a
Bournville	Cadbury	510	4.2	62.3	28.7	n/a
fruit & nut	Cadbury	495	5.3	61.1	27.4	n/a
Bournville Selection	Cadbury	470	3.4	66.3	22.9	n/a
Bournvita Powder		341	7.7	79.0	1.5	N
made up with whole milk		76.0	3.4	7.6	3.8	Tr
made up with semi-skimmed milk		58.0	3.5	7.6	1.6	Tr
Boursin						
au concombre	Van Den Berghs	236	8.0	4.0	21.0	n/a
au Roquefort	Van Den Berghs	243	8.5	4.0	21.5	n/a
aux olives	Van Den Berghs	234	8.0	3.5	21.0	n/a
with garlic	Van Den Berghs	413	7.3	2.7	41.5	n/a
with pepper	Van Den Berghs	421	7.4	1.2	43.0	n/a

All amounts given per 100g/100ml unless otherwise stated

Product	Brand	Calories kcal	Protein (g)	Carbo-hydrate (g)	Fat (g)	Dietary Fibre (g)
Bovril		169	38.0	2.9	0.7	nil
Boysenberries in Syrup	Libby	68.0	n/a	n/a	Tr	n/a
Braised Beef, canned	Tyne Brand	138	11.3	8.0	7.0	n/a
Bramley Apple Dessert	Mr Kipling	328	3.4	55.8	11.7	n/a
Bramley Apple Hot Cake	McVitie's	314	3.9	43.1	14.6	1.3
Bran						
natural	Boots	166	15.0	19.0	3.9	44.0
natural country	Jordans	190	15.0	27.0	n/a	4.0
Bran Buds	Kellogg's	290	13.0	52.0	3.0	22.0
Bran Fare	Weetabix	253	17.0	35.1	5.0	34.2
Bran Flakes	Kellogg's	318	10.2	69.3	1.9	17.3
Bran Oatcakes, each	Paterson's	54.0	n/a	n/a	1.8	n/a
	Vessen	57.0	1.5	7.8	2.1	0.9
Bran, wheat		206	14.1	26.8	5.5	39.6
Brandy: see Spirits						

Branston Fruity Sauce	Crosse & Blackwell	117	0.9	25.6	0.2	1.1
Branston Sandwich Pickle	Crosse & Blackwell	122	0.8	28.0	0.1	1.7
Branston Spicy Sauce	Crosse & Blackwell	115	1.0	23.9	0.7	1.3
Branston Sweet Pickle	Crosse & Blackwell	150	0.7	34.5	0.2	1.7
Brasilia Gourmet Sauce	Rakusen	80.0	n/a	n/a	2.7	n/a
Brawn		153	12.4	nil	11.5	nil
Brazil Nut Toffees, each	Trebor Bassett	28.0	0.2	3.0	1.7	n/a
Brazil Nuts		682	14.1	3.1	68.2	8.1
Brazil Roast	Granose	485	20.6	44.6	24.0	n/a
***Bread** (see also flavours)*						
brown		218	8.5	44.3	2.0	5.9
brown, toasted		272	10.4	56.5	2.1	7.1
currant		289	7.5	50.7	7.6	3.8

All amounts given per 100g/100ml unless otherwise stated

Product	Brand	Calories kcal	Protein (g)	Carbo-hydrate (g)	Fat (g)	Dietary Fibre (g)
currant, toasted		323	8.4	56.8	8.5	4.2
French stick		270	9.6	55.4	2.7	5.1
granary		235	9.3	46.3	2.7	6.5
malt		268	8.3	56.8	2.4	6.5
pitta, white		265	9.2	57.9	1.2	3.9
rye		219	8.3	45.8	1.7	5.8
wheatgerm		212	9.5	41.5	2.0	5.1
wheatgerm, toasted		271	12.1	53.2	2.6	6.5
white		235	8.4	49.3	1.9	3.8
white, fried in oil/lard		503	7.9	48.5	32.2	3.8
white, toasted		265	9.3	57.1	1.6	4.5
wholemeal		215	9.2	41.6	2.5	7.4
wholemeal, toasted		252	10.8	48.7	2.9	8.7
Bread Pudding		297	5.9	49.7	9.6	3.0
Bread Rolls, brown						
crusty		255	10.3	50.4	2.8	7.1
soft		268	10.0	51.8	3.8	6.4
Bread Rolls, white						

crusty		280	10.9	57.6	2.3	4.3
soft		268	9.2	51.6	4.2	3.9
Bread Rolls, wholemeal		241	9.0	48.3	2.9	8.8
Bread Sauce						
made with whole milk		150	4.1	10.9	10.3	0.6
made with semi-skimmed milk		128	4.2	11.1	7.8	0.6
Bread Sauce Mix	Colman's	316	8.3	n/a	1.0	n/a
	Knorr	372	11.1	67.5	8.3	2.1
Breadfruit, canned, drained		66.0	0.6	16.4	0.2	2.5
Breakaway, milk	Rowntree Mackintosh	519	6.6	68.0	26.4	n/a
plain	Rowntree Mackintosh	526	5.2	68.9	27.4	n/a
Breakfast Juice	Del Monte	38.0	0.5	9.4	Tr	n/a
Brie Cheese		319	19.3	Tr	26.9	nil
Brinjal Pickle	Sharwood	251	0.9	22.6	1.0	1.7
Broad Beans, boiled		48.0	5.1	5.6	0.8	5.4

All amounts given per 100g/100ml unless otherwise stated

Product	Brand	Calories kcal	Protein (g)	Carbohydrate (g)	Fat (g)	Dietary Fibre (g)
frozen, boiled		81.0	7.9	11.7	0.6	6.5
canned		77.0	5.9	13.0	0.5	5.2
Broccoli, boiled		24.0	3.1	1.1	0.8	2.3
Broccoli & Gruyere Soup	Baxters	56.0	2.0	4.7	3.3	0.9
Broccoli in Cheese Sauce	Findus Dinner Supreme	118	6.4	6.5	7.6	1.9
Broccoli Mix	Ross	41.0	2.3	9.0	0.5	2.3
Broccoli Spears, frozen premium choice	Findus	30.0	3.2	4.0	0.2	1.5
	Ross	24.0	2.9	4.1	0.7	2.6
1oz/28g	Birds Eye	7.0	1.0	1.5	Tr	n/a
Brown Ale, bottled		28.0	0.3	3.0	Tr	nil
Brown Bread: see Bread & also flavours						
Brown Lentils: see Lentils						
Brown Rice: see Rice						
Brown Sauce, bottled	Daddies	99.0	1.1	25.2	nil	0.7
		87.1	1.0	20.0	0.3	n/a

Brussels Pate	Delight	210	12.0	4.0	17.0	n/a
Brussels Sprouts, boiled						
frozen	Findus	35.0	2.9	3.5	1.3	2.6
1oz/28g	Birds Eye	27.0	4.0	2.7	Tr	4.1
premium choice	Ross	9.0	1.0	1.0	Tr	n/a
		35.0	4.1	6.6	0.5	3.2
Bubble & Squeak	Ross	119	1.6	14.4	6.7	1.3
Bubble Gum, per piece	Wrigley Hubba Bubba	11.2	n/a	n/a	n/a	n/a
Bumper Harvest Soups (Campbell's): *see flavours*						
Buns: *see flavours*						
Burgundy Cook-In-Sauce	Homepride	50.0	0.7	7.1	n/a	n/a
Burger Baps	Mothers Pride	255	9.2	43.6	4.4	2.5
Burger in a Bun Snackshot, per pack	Birds Eye	232	15.0	32.0	17.0	n/a
Burger Mix	Granose	455	28.0	32.5	31.0	n/a
Burger Relish	Daddies	90.0	1.9	21.4	Tr	n/a
Butter		737	0.5	Tr	81.7	nil

All amounts given per 100g/100ml unless otherwise stated

Product	Brand	Calories kcal	Protein (g)	Carbohydrate (g)	Fat (g)	Dietary Fibre (g)
unsalted	Kerrygold	720	n/a	n/a	n/a	n/a
all other brands	St Ivel	750	0.5	0.5	83.0	n/a
	St Ivel	740	0.5	0.5	81.0	n/a
Butter Beans, dried, boiled						
canned		103	7.1	18.4	0.6	5.2
		77.0	5.9	13.0	0.5	4.6
Butter Puffs	Crawfords	505	8.9	60.8	24.3	2.6
Buttercream Walnut Cake	Mr Kipling	400	5.2	50.9	20.9	n/a
Buttered Kipper Fillets	Birds Eye	220	17.5	nil	16.6	n/a
Butterfly Tops Cake Mix, per serving	Homepride Perfect	98.0	1.0	5.0	13.0	n/a
Buttermilk, cultured	Raines	40.0	4.3	5.5	0.1	nil
Buttermint Bonbons	Cravens	410	0.5	84.6	8.6	nil
Butterscotch Flavour Pouring Syrup	Lyle's	284	Tr	76.0	nil	Tr
Buttons, chocolate	Cadbury	520	7.7	58.7	29.9	n/a
white chocolate	Cadbury	520	8.5	59.5	29.2	n/a

Cabbage, average, raw		26.0	1.7	4.1	0.4	2.4
boiled		16.0	1.0	2.2	0.4	1.8
Caerphilly Cheese		375	23.2	0.1	31.3	nil
Cajun Sauce	Burgess	175	1.0	33.2	3.5	1.6
Calabrese: *see Broccoli*						
Calamari, Golden	Young's	228	11.4	23.1	10.4	1.0
Californian Crunchy Cereal	Jordans	395	8.0	62.8	14.2	7.0
Calippo Choc Bars, each						
lemon	Wall's	85.0	Tr	23.0	Tr	n/a
orange	Wall's	95.0	Tr	24.0	Tr	n/a

All amounts given per 100g/100ml unless otherwise stated

Product	Brand	Calories kcal	Protein (g)	Carbo-hydrate (g)	Fat (g)	Dietary Fibre (g)
Cambozola Cheese	St Ivel	466	13.5	Tr	43.5	nil
Camembert		297	20.9	Tr	23.7	nil
Candytots	Rowntree Mackintosh	388	0.7	96.5	2.6	n/a
Canellini Beans	Napolina	70.0	4.9	12.9	0.2	5.2
Cannelloni per pack	Birds Eye	415	25.0	43.0	17.0	n/a
	Mama Mia's	132	6.0	14.3	5.9	0.6
low calorie	Heinz Weight Watchers	68.0	2.9	9.5	2.0	1.7
Cannelloni Bistro Break	HP	102	5.2	11.3	4.0	2.9
Cannelloni Bolognese	Dolmio Ready Meals	143	6.1	10.9	8.6	n/a
Cannelloni Spinach & Ricotta	Dolmio Ready Meals	217	10.8	10.7	14.8	n/a
Cantonese Beef &						

Ginger with Special Noodles	Heinz	97.0	7.0	10.9	2.8	0.7
Cantonese Sweet & Sour Chicken Dish	Knorr	87.0	0.8	21.8	0.2	0.5
Cantonese Sweet & Sour Cook-In-Sauce	Homepride	129	0.3	29.7	n/a	n/a
Cantonese Sweet & Sour Pork Microwave Meal	Sharwood	157	5.8	20.2	5.7	1.2
Capelletti Milano	Dolmio Ready Meals	170	6.5	17.0	8.9	n/a
Cappuccino, instant	Nescafe Nestlé	386 394	10.6 14.2	62.8 52.0	10.3 14.3	nil nil
Cappuccino Vienetta	Wall's	140	2.0	15.0	8.5	n/a
Captain's Pie, per pack	Birds Eye MenuMaster	315	23.0	31.0	12.0	n/a
Captain's Quarter Pounder, each	Birds Eye MenuMaster	245	15.0	16.0	14.0	n/a

All amounts given per 100g/100ml unless otherwise stated

Product	Brand	Calories kcal	Protein (g)	Carbo- hydrate (g)	Fat (g)	Dietary Fibre (g)
Caramac	Rowntree Mackintosh	552	5.3	61.7	33.3	n/a
Caramel, per bar	Cadbury	245	2.9	30.6	12.9	n/a
Caramel & Walnut Cream Cake	McVitie's	317	3.5	36.9	17.6	0.7
Caramel Cakes, each	Cadbury	72.0	1.1	10.4	3.2	n/a
Caramel Flavour Milk Chocolate Coated Sandwich Wafers, diabetic	Boots	530	9.3	53.0	30.0	1.7
Caramel Granymels	Itona	385	0.8	69.0	13.2	n/a
Caramel Instant Chocolate Drink	Boots Shapers	356	16.0	58.0	8.3	4.2
Caramel Log	Tunnock's	472	4.2	64.3	24.0	n/a
Caramel Shortcake, each	Mr Kipling	162	1.1	19.4	9.1	n/a
Caramel Supreme	Eden Vale	127	3.9	21.3	3.5	n/a
Caramel Treats	Lyons	474	5.1	57.7	26.4	0.4

Caramel Wafers	Rowntree Mackintosh	463	4.6	68.6	20.8	n/a
	Tunnock's	454	4.6	68	20.1	n/a
Carbonara Pasta Sauce						
chilled	Dolmio	179	3.8	6.5	15.5	n/a
jar	Dolmio	131	1.6	4.5	11.8	n/a
Caribbean Chicken Stir Fry	Ross	99.0	6.0	13.1	3.1	1.4
Caribbean Crunchy Cereal	Holland & Barrett	390	12.0	60.0	12.0	14.0
Carnation	Nestlé	160	8.2	11.5	9.0	n/a
light	Nestlé	108	7.6	10.5	4.0	n/a
Carnation Slender Plan Bars						
apple & raisin	Nestlé	350	10.8	52.1	12.2	8.8
chocolate flavour	Nestlé	452	23.1	46.5	20.6	3.9
date & peanut	Nestlé	425	12.7	48.8	21.3	9.8
Carnation Slender Plan Drinks made with whole milk						
chocolate	Nestlé	229	11.0	27.9	8.2	0.1

All amounts given per 100g/100ml unless otherwise stated

Product	Brand	Calories kcal	Protein (g)	Carbohydrate (g)	Fat (g)	Dietary Fibre (g)
coffee	Nestlé	228	11.0	28.4	7.8	Tr
raspberry	Nestlé	228	11.0	28.5	7.8	Tr
strawberry	Nestlé	228	11.0	28.5	7.8	Tr
vanilla	Nestlé	230	11.0	29.0	7.8	Tr
made with semi-skimmed						
chocolate	Nestlé	166	11.3	28.3	0.8	0.1
coffee	Nestlé	165	11.4	28.9	0.4	Tr
raspberry	Nestlé	166	11.4	29.2	0.4	Tr
strawberry	Nestlé	166	11.4	29.2	0.4	Tr
vanilla	Nestlé	167	11.4	29.4	0.4	Tr
Carnation Slender Plan Fibre Bars						
apple & banana	Nestlé	385	4.0	63.8	12.6	5.7
apricot	Nestlé	364	5.7	53.4	14.2	11.7
plum	Nestlé	360	4.9	52.9	14.3	9.1
Carob Coated Fruit Bar, each	Granose	145	1.4	25.9	2.7	1.1
Carob Soya Milk	Granose	45.0	2.4	5.5	1.4	n/a
Carrot & Butter Bean Soup	Baxters	47.0	1.6	6.8	1.7	2.3

		259	2.8	46.8	7.5	1.3
Carrot Cake	California Cake & Cookie Co.					
Carrot Juice		24.0	0.5	5.7	0.1	N
Carrots						
old, raw		35.0	0.6	7.9	0.3	2.4
old, boiled		24.0	0.6	4.9	0.4	2.5
young, raw		30.0	0.7	6.0	0.5	2.4
young, boiled		22.0	0.6	4.4	0.4	2.3
frozen, boiled		22.0	0.4	4.7	0.3	2.3
canned		20.0	0.5	4.2	0.3	1.9
Carte D'Or Ice Cream (Wall's): see flavours						
Cartoons Cake Mix, made up, per serving, all flavours	Green's	64.0	1.0	12.0	2.0	n/a
Cashew Nuts, roasted, salted		611	20.5	18.8	50.9	3.2
Cashew Roast	Granose	502	20.1	43.2	26.8	8.4
Cassava, fresh, raw		142	0.6	36.8	0.2	1.6
baked		155	0.7	40.1	0.2	1.7
boiled		130	0.5	33.5	0.2	1.4

All amounts given per 100g/100ml unless otherwise stated

73

Product	Brand	Calories kcal	Protein (g)	Carbo-hydrate (g)	Fat (g)	Dietary Fibre (g)
Casserole Mixes (Colman's): *see flavours*						
Caster Sugar	Tate & Lyle	394	nil	99.9	nil	nil
Castle Orange Marmalade	Baxters	200	Tr	53	nil	0.8
Cauliflower, raw		34.0	3.6	3.0	0.9	1.8
boiled		28.0	2.9	2.1	0.9	1.6
frozen, boiled		20.0	2.0	2.0	0.5	1.2
Cauliflower & Broccoli in Cheese Sauce	Ross	72.0	4.5	4.4	4.7	1.5
Cauliflower Cheese	Findus Dinner	105	5.9	5.1	6.9	1.3
	Supreme	113	6.2	6.5	7.6	1.2
per pack	Birds Eye MenuMaster	410	18.0	33.0	24.0	n/a
Cauliflower Cheese Jackets, each	Birds Eye	375	16.0	47.0	15.0	n/a
Cauliflower Cheese Quarter Pounders, each	Birds Eye	220	7.0	17.0	14.0	n/a

74

Celeriac, raw		18.0	1.2	2.3	0.4	3.7
boiled		15.0	0.9	1.9	0.5	3.2
Celery, raw		7.0	0.5	0.9	0.2	1.1
boiled		8.0	0.5	0.8	0.3	3.2
Celery Burgers	Granose	153	9.0	22.0	3.0	n/a
Celery Soup, low calorie	Heinz Weight Watchers	22.0	0.6	3.2	0.7	0.4
Channa Dhal	Sharwood	140	5.0	13.9	7.6	2.7
Chapati flour, brown		333	11.5	73.7	1.2	N
white		335	9.8	77.6	0.5	N
Chapati, Paratha & Puri Mix	Sharwood	321	10.2	63.1	2.0	6.6
Chapatis, made with fat		328	8.1	48.3	12.8	N
made without fat		202	7.3	43.7	1.0	N
Chasseur Casserole Recipe Sauce	Knorr	71.0	1.6	10.3	2.9	n/a
Chasseur Sauce	Colman's	36.0	1.4	n/a	0.5	n/a
Cook-In-Sauce Classic	Homepride	47.0	1.2	9.4	n/a	n/a

All amounts given per 100g/100ml unless otherwise stated

Product	Brand	Calories kcal	Protein (g)	Carbo-hydrate (g)	Fat (g)	Dietary Fibre (g)
Cheddar & Onion Cottage Cheese	Eden Vale	122	12.0	1.8	7.5	n/a
Cheddar Cheese		412	25.5	0.1	34.4	nil
Cheddar-type Cheese, reduced fat		261	31.5	Tr	15.0	nil
Cheddar Cheese Golden Lights, per pack	Golden Wonder	111	1.3	15.8	5.1	n/a
Cheddar Cheese Potatoes & Sauce	Batchelors	341	9.1	70.5	4.5	n/a
Cheddar Cheese Savoury Pancakes	Findus	202	7.5	23.1	8.8	0.9
Cheddar Cheese Slices, processed	Kraft	326	22.0	1.0	26.0	n/a
Cheddar Style Cheese	Flora	395	24.5	Tr	33.0	n/a
Cheddar with Herbs & Garlic	St Ivel	410	25.4	0.5	34.3	n/a
Cheddarie Cheddar Cheese Spread	Kraft	280	15.0	7.0	21.0	n/a

Cheddars	McVitie's	247	11.0	49.9	32.8	1.9
Cheese: *see flavours*						
Cheese & Broccoli Pasta & Sauce	Batchelors	365	17.2	69.1	4.1	n/a
Cheese & Celery Dairy Spread, low fat	Boots Shapers	164	16.0	4.9	8.5	nil
Cheese & Chive Oatsters	Jordans	399	9.6	59.0	15.5	7.0
Cheese & Chives Dairy Spread, low fat	Boots Shapers	164	16.0	4.9	8.5	nil
Cheese & Ham Dairy Spread, reduced fat	Heinz Weight Watchers	169	15.7	3.8	10.1	nil
Cheese & Mustard Seed Rolls, each	Sunblest	152	6.6	22.8	3.8	1.3
Cheese & Onion Crisps, per pack thick & crunchy	Golden Wonder Golden Wonder	153 143	2.1 2.0	12.5 14.3	10.5 9.0	n/a n/a
Cheese & Onion Pastie	Ross	270	6.4	23.4	17.2	1.0

All amounts given per 100g/100ml unless otherwise stated

Product	Brand	Calories kcal	Protein (g)	Carbo-hydrate (g)	Fat (g)	Dietary Fibre (g)
Cheese & Onion Pizza	McCain Pizza Pantry	168	7.0	29.7	3.2	n/a
	McVitie's	177	7.7	25.4	5.6	1.5
	Ross	222	8.0	30.0	8.3	1.3
Cheese & Onion Ringos, per pack	Golden Wonder	85.0	1.7	13.3	3.0	n/a
Cheese & Onion Sandwich Biscuits	Nabisco	461	10.0	55.0	23.5	3.0
Cheese & Onion Sticks	Nabisco	538	14.6	37.5	37.5	1.1
Cheese & Tomato Bontos	McVitie's	224	8.3	32.8	7.2	1.4
Cheese & Tomato Pizza deep pan 5"	St Ivel	235	9.0	24.8	11.8	1.5
	McCain Pizza Pantry	222	8.9	24.5	10.5	n/a
French bread	Findus	164	6.9	28.3	3.4	n/a
French bread, reduced calorie	Findus	235	9.2	27.0	10.0	1.4
	Findus Lean Cuisine	190	10.0	26.3	5.0	1.4

individual, each	Heinz Weight Watchers	136	9.2	14.2	4.7	2.2
	Birds Eye / Gino Ginelli	270	10.0	32.0	12.0	n/a
	Ross	221	7.6	29.1	8.3	1.2
luxury, each	Birds Eye / Gino Ginelli	515	25.0	77.0	14.0	n/a
traditional	St Ivel	260	10.5	28.4	12.4	n/a
Cheese & Tomato Sticks	Nabisco	517	11.3	39.8	37.5	3.5
Cheese, Celery & Grape Salad	Boots Shapers	151	9.3	6.3	10.0	0.6
Cheese Cream Pasta Sauce, dry, as sold	Buitoni	447	20.3	35.4	25.0	0.6
Cheese Dairy Spread, low fat	Boots Shapers	164	16.0	4.9	8.5	nil
	Heinz Weight Watchers	180	16.2	4.4	10.8	nil
Cheese, Egg & Bacon Flan, each	Birds Eye	900	29.0	61.0	62.0	n/a
Cheese, Onion & Chive	Heinz Weight					

All amounts given per 100g/100ml unless otherwise stated

Product	Brand	Calories kcal	Protein (g)	Carbo-hydrate (g)	Fat (g)	Dietary Fibre (g)
Dairy Spread, reduced fat	Watchers	173	15.2	5.8	9.9	0.4
Cheese, Onion & Tomato Flan, each	Birds Eye	750	24.0	56.0	63.0	n/a
Cheese Puffs	Boots	507	7.0	63.0	27.0	n/a
Cheese Ritz Crackers	Jacob's	480	3.3	66.0	22.9	n/a
Cheese Sandwich	Nabisco	487	10.2	53.3	27.4	1.8
Cheese Sauce *made up with whole milk* *with semi-skimmed milk*		197 179	8.0 8.1	9.0 9.1	14.6 12.6	0.2 0.2
Cheese Sauce Packet Mix *made up with whole milk* *with semi-skimmed milk*		110 90	5.3 5.4	9.3 9.5	6.1 3.8	N N
Cheese Singles	Kraft	300	20.0	1.0	24.0	n/a
Cheese Spread, plain		276	13.5	4.4	22.8	nil
Cheese Spread Alternative triangles, each	Flora Flora	310 57.0	14.0 2.4	7.0 1.1	25.0 6.6	n/a n/a

Cheese Spread Triangles, each with ham, each	Delight	36.0	2.4	1.1	2.4	n/a
	Delight	35.0	2.3	1.1	2.4	n/a
Cheese Squares	Boots	519	4.3	57.0	32.0	n/a
Cheese Sticks	Nabisco	539	15.5	38.5	37.5	0.7
Cheese Supreme Deep Pan Pizza	McCain Pizza Perfection	212	11.0	29.6	6.3	n/a
Cheese, Tomato & Vegetable Pizza Slice	McCain Pizza Pantry	159	7.4	27.8	2.8	n/a
Cheeseburger, per pack	Birds Eye Snackshots	370	17.0	30.0	21.0	n/a
each	McDonald's	272	14.7	32.5	10.2	2.5
Cheesecake: see also flavours						
Cheesecake, frozen		242	5.7	33.0	10.6	0.9
Cheesecake Mix: see flavours						
Cheesecakes	Sunblest	494	4.8	51.4	29.9	1.5
Cheeselets	Peek Frean	472	10.6	48.6	27.4	2.7

All amounts given per 100g/100ml unless otherwise stated

Product	Brand	Calories kcal	Protein (g)	Carbo-hydrate (g)	Fat (g)	Dietary Fibre (g)
Cheesey Pasta, made up	Kraft	214	5.3	23.9	10.7	n/a
Cheesey Wotsits, per pack	Golden Wonder	115	2.0	11.8	7.0	n/a
Chelsea Buns		366	7.8	56.1	13.8	1.7
Cherries, raw		48.0	0.9	11.5	0.1	0.9
canned in syrup		71.0	0.5	18.5	Tr	0.6
glacé		251	0.4	66.4	Tr	0.9
Cherry & Almond Real Fruit Le Yogurt, stirred, low fat	Chambourcy	102	5.3	16.4	1.7	0.1
Cherry & Blackcurrant Sponge Pudding	Mr Kipling	418	3.6	74.3	13.8	n/a
Cherry & Raisin Malt Loaf	Sunblest	274	9.1	55.0	2.0	5.2
Cherry Bakewell	Lyons	404	3.4	66.3	15.8	1.2
each	Mr Kipling	202	2.0	31.0	8.5	n/a
Cherry Brandy		255	Tr	32.6	nil	nil
Cherry Carob Coated Fruit Snack Bar, each	Granose	168	3.0	31.3	3.5	2.3

Cherry Cheesecake	Chambourcy McVitie's	244 336	6.0 4.9	32.5 30.0	10.0 22.0	1.1 0.4
Cherry Cheesecake Mix, made up	Lyons Tetley	247	4.1	29.7	12.0	n/a
Cherry Muffins	Lyons	377	4.1	54.4	17.4	0.7
Cherry Pie Filling		82.0	0.4	21.5	Tr	0.4
Cherry Slices, each	Mr Kipling	129	1.4	16.9	6.7	n/a
Cherry Yogurt Fruit On Bottom low calorie	Classic Ski Ski Ski Diet	89.0 89.0 35.0	5.0 4.8 3.9	16.8 17.0 4.8	0.7 0.7 0.2	n/a n/a n/a
Cherryade	Corona R. Whites	25.0 20.0	n/a n/a	6.6 5.3	n/a n/a	n/a n/a
Cheshire Cheese		379	24.0	0.1	31.4	nil
Cheshire Cheese Wedge	St Ivel Shape	247	26.0	0.5	15.7	n/a
Chestnuts		170	2.0	36.6	2.7	4.1
Chewbas, each	Trebor Bassett	14.0	Tr	3.3	0.22	n/a

All amounts given per 100g/100ml unless otherwise stated

Product	Brand	Calories kcal	Protein (g)	Carbo-hydrate (g)	Fat (g)	Dietary Fibre (g)
Chewing Gum						
slab (spearmint, fruit, etc)	Wrigley	306	nil	2.4	nil	nil
sugar coated (arrowmint, etc)	Wrigley	352	nil	1.3	nil	nil
sugarfree slab (Orbit)	Wrigley	275	nil	nil	nil	nil
sugarfree coated	Wrigley	164	nil	nil	nil	nil
Chews (Trebor Bassett): see flavours						
Chick Pea Dhal	Sharwood	139	5.3	14.2	7.1	3.9
Chick Pea Spread: see Hummus						
Chick Peas, dried, boiled		121	8.4	18.2	2.1	4.3
canned		115	7.2	16.1	2.9	4.1
Chicken						
meat only, boiled		183	29.2	nil	7.3	nil
light meat, boiled		163	29.7	nil	4.9	nil
dark meat, boiled		204	28.6	nil	9.9	nil
meat only, roast		148	24.6	nil	5.4	nil
meat & skin, roasted		216	22.6	nil	14.0	nil
light meat, roasted		142	26.5	nil	4.0	nil

		kcal	Protein (g)	Carbohydrate (g)	Fat (g)	Fibre (g)
dark meat, roasted		155	23.1	nil	6.9	nil
leg quarter, roast, meat only		92.0	15.4	nil	3.4	nil
wing quarter, roast, meat only		74.0	12.4	nil	2.7	nil
breaded, fried in veg. oil		242	18.0	14.8	12.7	0.7
Chicken A La King Cook In The Pot Microwave Mix, as sold	Crosse & Blackwell	418	8.1	47.0	22.0	0.4
Chicken A L'Orange	Findus Lean Cuisine	106	9.0	13.3	1.8	0.8
Chicken & Asparagus Bake	Boots Shapers	102	9.4	10.0	3.0	2.0
Chicken & Bacon Scrunchy	Findus	246	6.7	22.9	14.2	0.6
Chicken & Bacon Savoury Pancakes	Findus	151	5.7	23.9	3.6	0.9
Chicken & Ham Lasagne, per pack	Birds Eye Healthy Options	355	31	39	9.5	n/a
Chicken & Ham Spread	Shippams	202	n/a	n/a	n/a	n/a
Chicken & Leek Soup, condensed	Campbell's	99.0	1.5	7.4	7.1	0.2

All amounts given per 100g/100ml unless otherwise stated

Product	Brand	Calories kcal	Protein (g)	Carbo-hydrate (g)	Fat (g)	Dietary Fibre (g)
Chicken & Mushroom, canned	Tyne Brand	107	3.7	6.3	7.4	n/a
Chicken & Mushroom Casserole, per pack	Birds Eye MenuMaster	160	18.0	6.0	7.0	n/a
Chicken & Mushroom Instant Pot Meal	Boots Shapers	381	14.0	66.0	8.6	n/a
Chicken & Mushroom Pasta & Sauce	Batchelors	346	15.3	72.9	1.3	n/a
Chicken & Mushroom Pie	Fray Bentos	177	9.1	16.3	8.9	n/a
Chicken & Mushroom Pie Filling	Fray Bentos	87.8	9.0	5.5	3.4	n/a
Chicken & Mushroom Savoury Pancake	Findus	161	5.5	22.0	5.7	1.0
Chicken & Mushroom Soup	Heinz	43.0	1.2	4.6	2.2	0.1
Chicken & Mushroom Toast Topper	Heinz	60.0	5.1	6.4	1.5	0.3

Chicken & Prawn Cantonese	Findus Lean Cuisine	102	7.0	10.6	3.4	1.9
Chicken & Rice Salad	Boots Shapers	103	7.3	11.0	3.6	0.9
Chicken & Sweetcorn Scrunchy	Findus	246	6.4	21.6	16.0	1.1
Chicken & Vegetable Broth with Rice	Campbell's Granny's Soups	46.0	0.3	7.6	1.6	0.4
Chicken & Vegetable pie canned	Tyne Brand	233	5.3	25.6	12.1	n/a
Golden Choice	Ross	251	7.5	25.3	13.8	1.1
Hungryman	Ross	254	8.3	19.8	16.1	0.8
Chicken & Vegetable Soup	Campbell's Main Course	46.0	2.1	6.1	1.4	0.9
	Heinz Big Soups	43.0	2.5	6.2	0.9	0.7
Chicken & Wholefood Salad with Rice	Boots	252	7.3	16.0	9.6	1.8
Chicken, Apple & Peach Salad, per pack	Boots	386	n/a	n/a	n/a	n/a

All amounts given per 100g/100ml unless otherwise stated

Product	Brand	Calories kcal	Protein (g)	Carbohydrate (g)	Fat (g)	Dietary Fibre (g)
Chicken Biryani	Batchelors Microchef Meal	102	7.0	15.3	1.8	n/a
per pack	Birds Eye MenuMaster	545	34.0	44.0	27.0	n/a
Chicken Broth	Baxters	32.0	0.8	5.4	0.9	0.7
Chicken Burgers, each	Birds Eye	160	7.0	9.0	11.0	n/a
Chicken Casserole canned per pack	Tyne Brand	100	4.2	7.1	6.3	n/a
	Birds Eye MenuMaster	345	23.0	41.0	11.0	n/a
Chicken Chasseur with Rice, per pack	Birds Eye MenuMaster	440	27.0	72.0	7.0	n/a
Chicken Chasseur Cook-In-Sauce	Homepride	48.0	1.0	8.2	n/a	n/a
Chicken Chasseur Cook In The Pot Dry Mix, as sold	Crosse & Blackwell	345	11.6	50.0	10.0	1.7
Chicken Chasseur						

All amounts given per 100g/100ml unless otherwise stated

Cooking Mix, as sold						
	Colman's	298	8.1	n/a	1.1	n/a
Chicken Curry						
	Batchelors Microchef Meal	143	6.8	21.9	3.1	n/a
	Boots Shapers	87.0	7.9	10.0	2.0	1.2
	Findus Dinner Supreme	127	6.0	18.1	3.4	0.8
per pack	Birds Eye MenuMaster	215	18.0	17.0	8.5	n/a
canned	Campbell's	87.0	4.9	9.7	3.2	1.5
	Tyne Brand	131	3.6	11.0	8.1	n/a
Chicken Curry with Rice						
	Batchelors Microchef Snack	87.0	4.0	12.0	2.7	n/a
	Vesta	99.0	2.9	20.3	1.2	n/a
per pack	Birds Eye	405	22.0	63.0	9.0	n/a
per pack	Heinz Lunchbowl	94.0	3.6	17.2	1.2	1.0
Chicken Curry Pancakes	Findus	162	5.6	23.3	5.2	1.2
Chicken Curry Snackshot, per pot	Birds Eye	215	12.0	33.0	4.5	n/a

All amounts given per 100g/100ml unless otherwise stated

Product	Brand	Calories kcal	Protein (g)	Carbo-hydrate (g)	Fat (g)	Dietary Fibre (g)
Chicken Dhansak	Shippams	96.0	n/a	n/a	n/a	n/a
Chicken Essence	Sharwood	50.0	12.4	0.2	n/a	n/a
Chicken Feasts, each cheese & ham mushroom	Birds Eye Birds Eye	280 245	14.0 16.0	16.0 15.0	18.0 14.0	n/a n/a
Chicken Fried Rice	Vesta	163	5.9	25.3	4.9	n/a
Chicken Gravy Granules, as sold	Brooke Bond	297	13.8	50.8	5.7	n/a
Chicken Grills in Natural Wheat Crumb, each	Birds Eye	200	11.0	13.0	13.0	n/a
Chicken Grillsteak	Ross	233	14.1	14.8	13.3	0.6
Chicken in a Bun Snackshot, per pack	Birds Eye	335.0	15.0	32.0	17.0	n/a
Chicken in Blackbean Sauce	Heinz	100	6.0	16.4	1.2	1.0
Chicken in Red Wine, per pack	Birds Eye Healthy Options	320	23.0	49.0	5.0	n/a

Chicken in Supreme Sauce with Vegetables	Heinz Weight Watchers	97.0	7.6	7.3	4.2	0.7
Chicken Kiev Platter, per pack	Birds Eye MenuMaster	785	24.0	26.0	28.0	n/a
Chicken Korma Bistro Break	HP	121	5.2	14.2	5.8	1.7
Chicken Korma Cook In The Pot Microwave Mix, as sold	Crosse & Blackwell	446	9.1	41.7	27.0	3.0
Chicken Korma with Pilau Rice per pack	Heinz Weight Watchers	84.0	4.9	12.7	1.5	1.0
	Birds Eye MenuMaster	555	27.0	55.0	27.0	n/a
Chicken Korma with Rice, per pack	Birds Eye Healthy Options	460	30.0	69.0	9.0	n/a
Chicken McNuggets (6)	McDonald's	276	20.5	12.3	16.4	0.4
Chicken Madras	Shippams	85.0	n/a	n/a	n/a	n/a

All amounts given per 100g/100ml unless otherwise stated

Product	Brand	Calories kcal	Protein (g)	Carbohydrate (g)	Fat (g)	Dietary Fibre (g)
Chicken Marengo with Rice	Heinz Weight Watchers	98.0	6.3	15.4	1.2	0.8
Chicken Masala	Shippams Vesta	121 94.0	n/a 3.7	n/a 18.1	n/a 1.3	n/a n/a
Chicken Meatballs in Gravy, canned	Campbell's	119	6.2	8.4	6.9	nil
Chicken Noodle & Sweetcorn Soup, instant, as sold	Boots Shapers	291	11.0	63.0	1.2	3.7
Chicken Noodle Soup, *dried*, *as sold* *dried, as served* **canned, low calorie**	Heinz Weight Watchers	329 20.0 20.0	13.8 0.8 1.2	60.9 3.7 3.3	5.0 0.3 0.2	4.3 0.2 0.4
Chicken Pate	Delight	218	12.5	4.0	17.0	n/a
Chicken Pie, original, each	Birds Eye	410	11.0	33.0	27.0	n/a
Chicken Provencale Cook In The Pot Dry Mix, as sold	Crosse & Blackwell	330	10.5	50.9	9.4	2.2
Chicken Quarter Pounders,						

each	Birds Eye	265	16.0	20.0	14.0	n/a
Chicken Ravioli in Mushroom Sauce	Heinz	69.0	11.9	2.9	1.1	0.8
Chicken Rice Soup, condensed	Campbell's	31.0	1.1	4.9	0.7	0.1
Chicken Roll, per slice	Delight	16.0	2.8	0.5	0.3	n/a
Chicken Satay with Peanut Sauce	Heinz	260	19.7	6.3	17.3	1.2
Chicken Savoury Rice	Batchelors	338	8.8	75.7	2.1	n/a
Chicken Seasoning Dry Sauce Mix, as sold	Colman's	314	11.0	n/a	1.4	n/a
Chicken Soup, canned, low calorie	Heinz Weight Watchers	21.0	0.8	2.2	1.0	0.1
Chicken Spread	Shippams	212	n/a	n/a	n/a	n/a
Chicken Stew, canned	Campbell's / Tyne Brand	79.0 / 75.0	4.2 / 3.3	9.8 / 5.9	2.7 / 2.2	0.9 / n/a
Chicken Stock Cubes	Knorr	324	11.6	23.3	21.3	0.5

All amounts given per 100g/100ml unless otherwise stated

Product	Brand	Calories kcal	Protein (g)	Carbo-hydrate (g)	Fat (g)	Dietary Fibre (g)
Chicken Stock Powder	Knorr	204	12.9	28.9	4.8	0.2
Chicken Supernoodles	Batchelors	474	7.4	56.2	26.0	n/a
Chicken Supreme	Birds Eye MenuMaster	250	22.0	10.0	14.0	n/a
	Boots Shapers	93.0	8.0	8.0	3.4	1.1
low calorie	Birds Eye MenuMaster	415	24.0	56.0	12.0	n/a
with rice, per pack	Vesta	115	3.6	17.6	3.8	n/a
Chicken Supreme Casserole Mix, as sold	Colman's	399	16.0	n/a	15.0	n/a
Chicken Supreme Cook-In-Sauce	Homepride	78.0	0.6	5.3	n/a	n/a
Chicken Tarragon Soup, condensed	Campbell's	93.0	2.6	7.6	5.8	0.2
Chicken Tikka Makhanwala with Pilau Rice, per pack	Birds Eye MenuMaster	490	26.0	54.0	20.0	n/a
Chicken Tikka Masala with	Findus Lean					

Turmeric Rice	Cuisine	98.0	6.0	14.1	1.9	1.6
Chicksticks, each	Birds Eye	65.0	3.0	5.5	3.5	n/a
Chicory, raw		11.0	0.5	2.8	0.6	0.9
Chilli & Garlic Marinade	Sharwood	90.0	2.9	17.7	1.0	1.6
Chilli & Garlic Sauce	Lea & Perrins	61.0	1.3	12.2	0.7	n/a
Chilli & Tomato Stir Fry Sauce	Sharwood	97.0	1.7	20.6	1.2	1.1
Chilli Bean & Beef Soup	Heinz	37.0	1.6	6.0	0.7	1.0
Chilli Bean Soup	Baxters	40.0	1.7	8.2	0.3	1.7
Chilli Beanfeast	Batchelors	341	22.3	57.5	4.0	n/a
Chilli Beans		70.0	4.9	12.2	0.5	3.9
Chilli Chinese Pouring Sauce						
hot	Sharwood	120	0.5	29.4	0.6	1.3
sweet	Sharwood	177	0.6	44.4	0.8	1.5
Chilli Con Carne, canned	Campbell's	108	6.2	12.7	3.5	2.9
	Old El Paso	118	n/a	n/a	n/a	n/a
	Tyne Brand	120	9.2	6.6	6.5	n/a

All amounts given per 100g/100ml unless otherwise stated

Product	Brand	Calories kcal	Protein (g)	Carbo-hydrate (g)	Fat (g)	Dietary Fibre (g)
Chilli Con Carne Casserole Mix	Colman's Crosse & Blackwell	303	n/a	8.7	1.9	n/a
		330	12.4	45.0	11.2	3.6
Chilli Con Carne Microchef Snack	Batchelors	76.0	5.6	10.0	1.8	n/a
Chilli Con Carne with American Rice	Findus Lean Cuisine	98.0	5.7	14.4	1.9	1.6
Chilli Con Carne with Rice, per pack	Birds Eye MenuMaster	380	19	66	6	n/a
	Birds Eye Healthy Options	425	21.0	85.0	2.5	n/a
	Heinz Lunchbowl	100	6.3	15.2	1.5	2.9
Chilli Dip, per pack	Kavli	350	6.9	6.0	33.3	n/a
Chilli Dip & Snack	Boots Shapers	483	17.9	61.2	20.0	22.8

						N
Chilli Peppers red, raw		26.0	1.8	4.2	0.3	N
green, raw		20.0	2.9	0.7	0.6	N
Chilli Sauce	HP	124	1.5	27.8	0.8	n/a
Chilli Seasoning Dry Sauce Mix, as sold	Colman's	328	9.2	n/a	3.9	n/a
Chilli with Kidney Beans Sauce	Colman's	187	2.1	n/a	0.5	n/a
China Fruit Salad in Syrup	Libby	70.0	n/a	n/a	Tr	n/a
Chinese Bean Salad	Batchelors	139	8.2	22.6	1.7	n/a
Chinese Chicken & Prawn Foo Young Stir Fry	Ross	77.0	5.5	12.3	1.4	1.8
Chinese Chicken Flavour Instant Noodles	Sharwood	433	10.2	56.0	17.7	2.3
Chinese Chicken Fried Savoury Rice	Batchelors	376	11.4	69.6	7.7	n/a
Chinese Chicken Snackshot, per pot	Birds Eye	225	13.0	38.0	3.5	n/a

All amounts given per 100g/100ml unless otherwise stated

Product	Brand	Calories kcal	Protein (g)	Carbohydrate (g)	Fat (g)	Dietary Fibre (g)
Chinese Chicken Stir Fry	Ross	80.0	7.3	11.9	1.1	1.8
Chinese Chicken with Rice, per pack	Birds Eye MenuMaster	345	22.0	56.0	5.0	n/a
Chinese Curry Flavour Instant Noodles	Sharwood	442	9.8	55.8	19.2	3.1
Chinese Fried Savoury Rice	Batchelors	371	9.5	70.1	7.8	n/a
Chinese Mixed Vegetables	Heinz	35.0	1.6	6.4	0.3	2.3
Chinese Mushroom, dried		284	10.0	59.9	1.8	Tr
Chinese Noodle Soup	Baxters	34.0	1.1	6.7	0.4	0.5
Chinese Pouring Sauces (Sharwood): *see flavours*						
Chinese Prawns Stir Fry	Ross	53.0	3.1	10.5	0.6	1.7
Chinese Sauce Mixes (Sharwood): *see flavours*						
Chinese Sizzling Prawns Stir Fry	Ross	39.0	3.3	8.2	0.3	2.5
Chinese Spare Rib Sauces (Sharwood): *see flavours*						

Chinese Special Rice	Ross	116	4.0	25.4	0.3	1.0
Chinese Spring Rolls	Ross	121	4.3	21.2	2.6	1.1
Chinese Style Beanfeast	Batchelors	313	30.9	38.0	5.2	n/a
Chinese Style Supernoodles	Batchelors	474	7.4	56.2	26.0	n/a
Chinese Sweet & Sour Chicken Soup	Campbell's	38.0	1.1	7.3	0.7	0.3
Chinese Sweet & Sour Chicken with Vegetables Soup	Heinz	40.0	2.0	6.6	0.6	0.4
Chinese Sweet & Sour Cook-In-Sauce	Homepride	83.0	0.5	18.4	n/a	n/a
Chinese Sweet & Sour Fried Savoury Rice	Batchelors	346	8.7	67.6	6.4	n/a
Chinese Sweet & Sour Pork Microwaveable Snack	Campbell's	149	4.0	18.2	6.7	0.5
Chinese Sweet & Sour Pork Stir Fry	Ross	78.0	4.5	12.8	1.6	1.4

All amounts given per 100g/100ml unless otherwise stated

Product	Brand	Calories kcal	Protein (g)	Carbo-hydrate (g)	Fat (g)	Dietary Fibre (g)
Chinese Tofu	Granose	60.0	2.5	4.0	4.0	0.9
Chinese Tomato & Noodle Soup, instant, as sold	Knorr	348	6.3	66.4	8.2	4.0
Chip Shop Chips	Ross	87.0	2.3	21.1	0.2	2.0
Chip Shop Fish (Ross): see flavours						
Chip Shop Mush Peas	Ross	103	7.5	23.6	0.2	5.7
Chippy Chips	McCain	91.0	2.4	20.1	0.1	1.6
Chips						
crinkle cut, frozen, fried		290	3.6	33.4	16.7	2.2
French fries, retail		280	3.3	34.0	15.5	2.1
homemade, fried		189	3.9	30.1	6.7	2.2
retail		239	3.2	30.5	12.4	2.2
straight cut, frozen, fried		273	4.1	36.0	13.5	2.4
Chips, microwave		221	3.6	32.1	9.6	2.9
crinkle cut	McCain	208	3.2	27.7	9.4	2.0
straight cut	McCain	223	3.2	28.5	10.7	2.05
Chips, oven		162	3.2	29.8	4.2	2.0

beefeater	Ross	147	3.1	24.6	5.0	2.2
crinkles	McCain	155	2.0	27.5	4.1	n/a
straight	McCain	157	1.9	26.7	4.7	n/a
wedges	McCain	154	1.9	26.9	4.3	1.5
	McCain	126	1.8	22.2	3.3	n/a
Chips, 3-Way Cook	Findus	107	2.2	17.9	3.0	2.2
Choc 'n' Nut Cornetto, each	Wall's	210	3.0	25.0	12.0	n/a
Choc 'n' Nut Ice Cream	Wall's Gino Ginelli Tubs	120	2.5	14.0	6.5	n/a
cup	Wall's	170	2.5	16.0	11.0	n/a
Choc 'n' Nut Supermousse, each	Birds Eye	150	3.0	16.0	9.0	n/a
Choc Bars (Wall's): *see flavours*						
Choc Chip & Hazelnut Cookies	McVitie's	504	5.4	65.2	24.3	2.0
Choc Chip 'n' Nut Cookies	Huntley & Palmer	438	5.4	62.8	25.5	1.7

All amounts given per 100g/100ml unless otherwise stated

Product	Brand	Calories kcal	Protein (g)	Carbo- hydrate (g)	Fat (g)	Dietary Fibre (g)
Choc Chip & Orange Cookies	McVitie's	501	5.3	65.8	23.8	2.0
Choc Chip Harvest Chewy Bar, each	Quaker	112	1.5	17.3	4.0	0.8
Choc Chip Oaties	Crawfords	492	6.1	66.8	21.9	2.6
Choc Ices: *see flavours*						
Choc Ripple Ice Cream	Lyons Maid	98.0	2.0	14.2	3.7	n/a
Chococino Hot Chocolate Drink	Rowntree	437	12.3	61.0	16.0	0.6
Chocolate: *see flavours*						
Chocolate & Fruit Ostlers	Lyons	454	5.8	62.1	22.0	5.4
Chocolate & Nut Crunch 'n' Slim	Crookes Healthcare	440	10.5	53.0	22.0	11.5
Chocolate & Orange Royale	McVitie's	286	5.6	27.5	17.1	0.2
Chocolate & Vanilla Swiss Roll	Lyons	440	3.5	57.0	23.6	0.7
Chocolate Bar Cake	McVitie's	377	4.8	53.8	14.9	1.3

Chocolate Biscuits, full-coated						
		524	5.7	67.4	27.6	2.1
Chocolate Blancmange	Brown & Polson	335	2.1	84.4	1.1	n/a
Chocolate Brownie Mix, made up, per serving	Green's	79.0	2.0	13.0	3.0	n/a
Chocolate Buttercream Shorties, each	Mr Kipling	134	1.3	15.8	7.7	n/a
Chocolate Cake	Cadbury	358	4.6	55.7	14.5	0.5
Chocolate Carmelle Mix, made up, per serving	Homepride	185	5.0	27.0	6.0	n/a
Chocolate Chip Solar	McVitie's	472	6.7	56.8	24.1	2.2
Chocolate Chip & Hazelnut Cookies	Boots	506	5.8	59.0	5.8	2.9
Chocolate Chip Cookie	California Cake & Cookie Co.	452	4.7	59.7	23.2	0.8
	Boots	476	6.2	62.0	26.0	2.5
diabetic						
Chocolate Chip Cookie Mix, made up, per serving	Green's	109	1.0	14.0	6.0	n/a

All amounts given per 100g/100ml unless otherwise stated

103

Product	Brand	Calories kcal	Protein (g)	Carbo-hydrate (g)	Fat (g)	Dietary Fibre (g)
Chocolate Chip Ginger Mini Cookies	Boots	462	4.5	68.0	21.0	2.1
Chocolate Chip Loaf	Sunblest	315	10.0	54.9	6.1	2.0
Chocolate Chip Muffin	California Cake & Cookie Co.	330	5.8	44.9	15.3	0.9
Chocolate Choice Dessert	Eden Vale	114	3.4	18.0	3.6	n/a
Chocolate Coated Apricot & Sultana Flapjack	Boots	477	6.0	56.0	27.0	3.1
Chocolate Coated Apricot Cereal Bar	Boots	411	5.5	63.0	17.0	3.4
Chocolate Coated Cereal & Hazelnut Bar	Boots	418	5.8	55.0	21.0	4.6
Chocolate Coated Fruit & Nut Flapjack	Boots	482	6.2	57.0	27.0	3.2
Chocolate Coated Ginger & Pear Bar	Boots	344	1.8	64.0	12.0	2.3

Chocolate Coated Raisin Bar	Boots	454	6.0	57.0	6.0	3.3
Chocolate Coffee Brownie Mix, made up, per serving	Homepride Simply Delicious	157	1.6	24.9	5.7	n/a
Chocolate Continental Roll	Lyons	372	4.2	58.7	15.0	0.9
Chocolate Cool Top Mix, made up, per serving	Homepride	198	3.0	30.0	7.0	n/a
Chocolate Cream, per bar	Cadbury	210	1.6	37.1	7.2	n/a
Chocolate Creme De Creme Ice Cream Cup, each	Lyons Maid	176	3.5	21.9	8.8	n/a
Chocolate Crusha	Burgess	187	nil	44.8	nil	nil
Chocolate Cup Cakes	Lyons	338	2.2	77.0	4.2	0.5
Chocolate Dairy Dessert	St Ivel Fiendish Feet	86.0	3.7	14.9	1.7	n/a
Chocolate Dairy Ice Cream	Boots Shapers	130	3.2	18.0	5.5	Tr
Chocolate Dairy Toffees, each	Trebor Bassett	45.0	0.3	5.7	2.6	n/a
Chocolate Dessert, made up						

All amounts given per 100g/100ml unless otherwise stated

Product	Brand	Calories kcal	Protein (g)	Carbo-hydrate (g)	Fat (g)	Dietary Fibre (g)
with whole milk, per serving	Bird's	161	5.5	19.6	6.3	n/a
Chocolate Digestive Bars	McVitie's	513	6.5	63.0	26.0	2.2
Chocolate Digestives: *see Digestive Biscuits*						
Chocolate Fancies	Lyons	488	5.3	52.6	29.9	0.3
Chocolate Flavour Dessert Mix, diabetic	Boots	132	3.2	15.5	6.3	Tr
Chocolate Flavour Sandwich Wafers, diabetic	Boots	497	12.0	56.0	25.0	2.9
Chocolate Fool Mix, made up	Lyons Tetley	216	4.7	24.1	10.9	n/a
Chocolate Freddie Mix, made up, per serving	Homepride	58.0	1.0	10.0	2.0	n/a
Chocolate Fruit & Nut Crunch	Mornflake	400	12.0	60.0	9.5	14.0
Chocolate, Fruit & Nut Slices, each	Mr Kipling	150	2.5	19.2	7.5	n/a
Chocolate Fudge, each	Trebor Bassett	43.0	Tr	6.2	2.1	n/a

Chocolate Fudge Brownie Mix, made up, per serving	Homepride Simply Delicious	164	2.0	24.5	6.4	n/a
Chocolate Fudge Cake	Lyons	423	3.8	54.4	22.6	0.6
	Mr Kipling	382	5.2	61.9	14.3	n/a
Chocolate Fudge Cake Mix, made up, per serving	Homepride Simply Delicious	122	1.0	21.4	3.6	n/a
Chocolate Fudge Dessert	Mr Kipling	412	3.5	57.7	20.2	n/a
Chocolate Fudge Slices, each	Mr Kipling	135	1.1	20.6	5.9	n/a
Chocolate Gateau Mix, made up, per serving	Green's	291	3.0	43.0	13.0	n/a
Chocolate Hob Nobs	McVitie's	497	6.3	62.8	24.3	3.7
Chocolate Homewheat	McVitie's	507	6.5	64.8	24.3	2.5
Chocolate Ice Cream	Lyons Maid	91.0	2.0	11.4	4.2	n/a
Chocolate Instant Whip, made up, per serving	Bird's	140	4.3	20.0	5.2	n/a
Chocolate Jaspers	McVitie's	506	6.0	64.7	24.5	2.7

All amounts given per 100g/100ml unless otherwise stated

Product	Brand	Calories kcal	Protein (g)	Carbo- hydrate (g)	Fat (g)	Dietary Fibre (g)
Chocolate Limes	Cravens	402	0.1	91.8	4.9	nil
Chocolate Lovely Tub Dessert, each	Birds Eye	235	4.0	22.0	15.0	n/a
Chocolate M & Ms: see M & Ms						
Chocolate Malted Food Drink low fat instant	Horlicks Horlicks	358 390	8.7 11.0	79.3 75.0	3.1 7.1	n/a n/a
Chocolate Microbake Mix, made up, per serving	Homepride	224	4.0	38.0	6.0	n/a
Chocolate Midi Rolls	Lyons	323	4.2	61.7	8.3	1.3
Chocolate Mini Rolls, each	Cadbury	117	1.4	15.6	5.8	n/a
Chocolate Mint Cool Top Mix, made up, per serving	Homepride	197	2.0	25.0	10.0	n/a
Chocolate Mint Cracknel	Cravens	438	0.5	82.9	12.0	nil
Chocolate Mint Creams, each	Trebor Bassett	37.0	Tr	7.3	1.2	n/a
Chocolate Mousse		139	4.0	19.9	5.4	N

Chocolate Muffins	Lyons	424	6.5	51.1	22.9	0.9
Chocolate Nesquik	Nestlé	371	3.1	83.4	2.8	0.8
made up with whole milk	Nestlé	171	7.1	18.5	8.1	0.1
with semi-skimmed milk	Nestlé	134	7.1	18.5	4.0	0.1
ready to drink	Nestlé	90.0	3.3	11.3	3.5	Tr
Chocolate Nut Spread		549	6.0	60.5	33.0	0.8
Chocolate Nut Sundae		278	3.0	34.2	15.3	0.1
Chocolate Oliver Biscuits	Fortts	359	6.5	69.5	23.9	3.9
Chocolate Orange Cool Top Mix, made up, per serving	Homepride	178	1.5	25.0	8.0	n/a
Chocolate Orange Fudge Cake Mix, made up, per serving	Homepride Simply Delicious	124	0.9	21.0	4.0	n/a
Chocolate Perkin	Tunnock's	506	7.5	62.0	25.9	n/a
Chocolate Praline Yogurt	Alpine Ski	94.0	5.5	16.8	1.0	n/a
Chocolate Ripple Dairy Ice Cream	Lyons Maid Napoli	96.0	2.1	14.0	3.5	n/a
Chocolate Ripple Ice Cream,	Heinz Weight					

All amounts given per 100g/100ml unless otherwise stated

Product	Brand	Calories kcal	Protein (g)	Carbo-hydrate (g)	Fat (g)	Dietary Fibre (g)
low calorie	Watchers	72.0	1.8	8.7	2.6	nil
Chocolate Roll	Cadbury	382	5.0	52.2	18.4	n/a
	Lyons	370	4.5	53.9	16.6	1.2
jam & vanilla	Lyons	322	4.2	61.5	8.3	1.4
Chocolate Sandwich	Lyons	371	4.1	53.0	17.5	0.9
Chocolate Slices	Lyons	423	4.4	57.2	21.2	0.5
Chocolate Sponge Pudding	Heinz	302	2.6	51.2	9.6	0.6
Chocolate Sponge Pudding Mix, made up	Homepride	209	3.5	35	6.0	n/a
Chocolate Supreme	Eden Vale	134	3.3	21.0	4.7	n/a
Chocolate Swiss Roll, boxed	Mr Kipling	328	4.3	53.0	12.5	n/a
Chocolate Truffle Cheesecake	McVitie's	381	6.1	34.3	24.5	0.4
Chocolate Vanilla Ice Cream	Delight	155	4.0	23.1	5.8	n/a
Chocolate Vienetta	Wall's	140	2.0	15.0	8.5	n/a
Chocolate Yogurt	St Ivel Fiendish					

	Feet	96.0	5.0	16.5	1.2	n/a
Chocolite Drink, low fat, as sold	Rowntree	371	17.2	67.0	3.8	0.9
no sugar added, as sold	Rowntree	351	24.2	56.0	3.4	1.2
Chocolova	McVitie's	370	3.3	46.5	19.0	Tr
Choice Grain Cracker	Jacob's	390	7.7	64.9	12.8	3.2
Choice Wholemeal Biscuits	McVitie's	481	7.6	66.5	19.9	6.5
Chomp, per bar	Cadbury	115	1.4	16.9	5.1	n/a
Chop Suey Sauce & Vegetables Stir Fry	Uncle Ben's	25.0	0.6	4.5	0.5	n/a
Chop Suey Stir Fry Sauce	Sharwood	75.0	0.7	14.6	1.5	0.2
Chopped Chilli Tomatoes	Napolina	16.0	1.2	3.0	Tr	1.0
Chopped Curry Tomatoes	Napolina	17.0	1.4	2.9	Tr	1.0
Chopped Ham & Pork, canned		275	14.4	1.4	23.6	0.3
Chopped Tomatoes	Napolina	14.0	1.2	2.5	Tr	1.0
Chopped Tomatoes with herbs	Napolina	15.0	1.2	2.5	Tr	1.0

All amounts given per 100g/100ml unless otherwise stated

Product	Brand	Calories kcal	Protein (g)	Carbo-hydrate (g)	Fat (g)	Dietary Fibre (g)
Chow Mein	Batchelors Microchef Snack	63.0	4.1	11.1	0.6	n/a
	Vesta	105	4.6	18.5	1.9	n/a
low calorie	Heinz Weight Watchers	70.0	3.3	9.6	2.0	2.0
Chow Mein Mix	Ross	46.0	1.9	10.8	0.4	2.1
Christmas Dundee Cake	McVitie's	366	5.6	63.4	10.2	5.0
Christmas Pudding, recipe retail		291	4.6	49.5	9.7	1.3
		329	3.0	56.3	11.8	1.7
Chunky Chicken, canned						
country style	Shippams	171	n/a	n/a	n/a	n/a
curry	Shippams	121	n/a	n/a	n/a	n/a
Spanish style	Shippams	153	n/a	n/a	n/a	n/a
supreme	Shippams	159	n/a	n/a	n/a	n/a
Chunky Chicken in Curry Mayonnaise Sandwich Maker	Shippams	206	n/a	n/a	n/a	n/a
Chunky Chicken in						

Mayonnaise Sandwich Maker	Shippams	213	n/a	n/a	n/a	n/a
Chunky Chips	McCain	127	2.9	25.0	2.4	n/a
	Ross	118	2.4	21.9	3.0	1.6
Chunky Choc Ice, each	Wall's	160	2.0	15.0	10.0	n/a
Chunky Dark Choc Ice, each	Wall's	160	2.0	15.0	11.0	n/a
Chutney: *see flavours*						
Cider, dry		36.0	Tr	2.6	nil	nil
sweet		42.0	Tr	4.3	nil	nil
vintage		101	Tr	7.3	nil	nil
low alcohol	Strongbow	16.0	n/a	n/a	n/a	n/a
Citrus Fruit Drink	Boots Shapers	0.3	Tr	nil	nil	nil
Citrus Fruit Fool	Boots Shapers	121	2.5	6.1	9.8	n/a
Citrus Fruit Yogurt	Boots Shapers	44.0	4.4	6.8	0.1	Tr
Classic Bean Salad	Batchelors	108	5.1	21.4	0.8	n/a
Classic Chinese Marinade	Sharwood	113	1.8	16.1	4.8	1.0
Classic Chocolate Cake	Lyons	456	5.9	50.0	27.2	0.6

All amounts given per 100g/100ml unless otherwise stated

Product	Brand	Calories kcal	Protein (g)	Carbohydrate (g)	Fat (g)	Dietary Fibre (g)
Classic Rolls	Lyons	425	5.0	60.0	21.8	0.6
Classic Selection	Lyons	473	5.1	56.3	26.8	0.5
Classico Dark Choc Ice	Lyons Maid	143	1.6	14.3	9.1	n/a
Classico Milk Choc Ice	Lyons Maid	148	1.8	14.5	9.6	n/a
Classico Salad Dressing	Napolina	558	0.4	5.4	56.0	n/a
Clementines, flesh only		37	0.9	8.7	nil	1.2
Cloudy Lemonade	Boots Shapers	0.2	Tr	nil	nil	nil
Clover	Dairy Crest	682	0.8	1.2	75.0	nil
extra lite	Dairy Crest	390	7.8	0.5	39.6	nil
lightly salted	Dairy Crest	682	0.8	1.2	75.0	nil
Club Biscuits (Jacob's): *see flavours*						
Club Soda	Cantrell & Cochrane	nil	nil	nil	nil	nil
Club Tonic	Cantrell & Cochrane	25.5	nil	6.8	nil	nil

Coca-Cola		39.0	Tr	10.5	nil	nil
Cock-a-Leekie Soup	Baxters	22.0	0.5	3.9	0.6	0.5
Cockles, boiled		48.0	17.2	Tr	2.0	nil
Cocktail Cherries	Burgess	247	0.3	61.4	nil	0.9
Cocktail Dressing For Seafood & Salads	Crosse & Blackwell Waistline	146	1.0	14.4	8.9	0.3
Coco Pops	Kellogg's	380	5.0	87.0	1.0	1.0
Cocoa Powder		312	18.5	11.5	21.7	12.1
made up with whole milk		76.0	3.4	6.8	4.2	0.2
made up with semi-skimmed milk		57.0	3.5	7.0	1.9	0.2
Coconut, creamed		669	6.0	7.0	68.8	N
desiccated		604	5.6	6.4	62.0	13.7
Coconut Bar Cake	McVitie's	357	5.7	51.3	14.4	2.3
Coconut Biscuits	Huntley & Palmer	500	5.1	55.6	30.1	6.3
Coconut Cookies	Huntley &					

All amounts given per 100g/100ml unless otherwise stated

Product	Brand	Calories kcal	Protein (g)	Carbohydrate (g)	Fat (g)	Dietary Fibre (g)
Coconut Cool Top Mix, made up, per serving	Palmer	481	4.8	54.5	28.5	5.8
Coconut Crunch Cake	Homepride	194	1.5	23.0	10.4	n/a
Coconut Crunch Cake	Lyons	501	4.3	52.9	31.8	1.8
Coconut Fruit Snack Bar, each	Granose	102	2.2	15.2	3.7	1.7
Coconut Macaroons, each	Mr Kipling	106	1.0	14.9	5.0	n/a
Coconut Mallows	Peek Frean	390	4.0	68.5	13.0	2.4
Coconut Oil		899	Tr	nil	99.9	nil
Coconut Soya Milk	Granose	71.0	3.5	5.8	3.8	n/a
Cod & Prawn Crepe	Ross Recipe Meal	146	9.2	13.4	6.4	0.6
Cod & Prawn Pie	Ross Recipe Meal	132	4.6	11.4	7.8	0.5
Cod Crumble	Ross Recipe Meal	192	9.8	14.4	10.8	0.6
Cod, dried, salted, boiled		138	32.5	nil	0.9	nil
Cod Fillet Fish Fingers, grilled, each	Birds Eye	50.0	3.5	5.0	2.0	n/a
	Findus	63.0	3.8	5.0	3.1	Tr

Cod Fillets						
baked		96.0	21.4	nil	1.2	nil
poached		94.0	20.9	nil	1.1	nil
	Ross Chip Shop	230	10.5	14.3	14.7	0.5
	Ross Fish Shop	76.0	17.4	nil	0.7	n/a
breaded	Ross Fish Shop	119	12.7	17.0	0.3	0.7
natural crumb	Ross	200	12.0	14.1	10.9	0.6
Cod Fish Cakes in Crispy Crunch Crumb, each	Birds Eye	80.0	4.5	8.5	3.5	n/a
Cod Fish Fingers						
each	Birds Eye	45.0	3.0	2.0	4.0	n/a
jumbo	Ross Chip Shop	247	10.2	13.8	17.1	0.7
oven crispy, each	Birds Eye	80.0	3.5	5.0	5.5	n/a
prime, each	Birds Eye	45.0	3.0	2.0	4.0	n/a
wholemeal breadcrumbs, each	Birds Eye	50.0	3.0	3.5	2.5	n/a
Cod in Wine & Herb Sauce, per pack	Birds Eye Healthy Options	280	22.0	30.0	9.0	n/a
Cod in Wine &	Birds Eye					

All amounts given per 100g/100ml unless otherwise stated

Product	Brand	Calories kcal	Protein (g)	Carbohydrate (g)	Fat (g)	Dietary Fibre (g)
Mushroom Sauce, per pack	Healthy Options	245	25.0	21.0	7.0	n/a
Cod Liver Oil		899	Tr	nil	99.9	nil
Cod Mornay, per pack	Birds Eye	480	30.0	31.0	27.0	n/a
	MenuMaster					
Cod Roe, hard, fried	Birds Eye	202	20.9	3.0	11.9	0.1
Cod Steak						
in butter sauce	Findus	110	11.0	3.8	5.6	Tr
	Ross	88.0	10.0	3.0	4.0	0.1
per pack	Birds Eye	160	16.0	10.0	6.5	n/a
in cheese sauce, per pack	MenuMaster	170	20.0	7.0	7.0	n/a
	Birds Eye	160	18.0	7.5	6.5	n/a
in mushroom sauce, per pack	MenuMaster	155	17.0	11.0	5.0	n/a
in parsley sauce, per pack	Findus	104	10.7	3.6	5.2	Tr
	Ross	89.0	10.4	2.9	4.0	0.1

		214	11.8	14.0	12.3	0.5
Cod Steaklets in Battercrisp, oven baked, each	Findus					
Cod Steaks						
grilled		95.0	20.8	nil	1.3	nil
in batter, fried in oil		199	19.6	nil	10.3	0.3
	Ross Chip Shop	204	11.1	11.7	12.7	0.4
crispy crunch crumb, each	Birds Eye	220	14.0	13.0	13.0	n/a
harvest crumb, each	Birds Eye	201	12.0	17.0	11.0	n/a
natural, each	Birds Eye	80.0	18.0	nil	0.5	n/a
natural crumb	Ross	200	10.6	16.3	10.6	0.7
oven crispy, each	Birds Eye	230	12.0	13.0	15.0	n/a
waterlight, each	Birds Eye	195	12.0	12.0	11.0	n/a
wholemeal crumb, each	Birds Eye	195	14.0	13.0	10.0	n/a
Coffee, infusion, 5 minutes		2.0	0.2	0.3	Tr	nil
instant		100	14.6	11.0	Tr	nil
Coffee Club Biscuits	Jacob's	505	5.6	63.1	27.3	0.8
Coffee Creams	Peek Frean	480	5.1	72.5	20.6	2.0

All amounts given per 100g/100ml unless otherwise stated

Product	Brand	Calories kcal	Protein (g)	Carbohydrate (g)	Fat (g)	Dietary Fibre (g)
Coffee Flavour Milk Chocolate, diabetic	Boots	450	9.6	46.0	32.0	4.0
Coffee Gateau Mix, made up, per serving	Green's	296	3.0	46.0	12.0	n/a
Coffee-Mate, per 4.5g tsp						
regular	Carnation	25.0	0.1	2.5	1.6	nil
lite	Carnation	19.0	Tr	3.0	0.7	nil
Coffee Swiss Gateau	Cadbury	384	4.5	55.2	17.6	n/a
Cola Refresher	Trebor Bassett	7.0	n/a	1.7	0.1	n/a
Coleslaw						
canned	Heinz	134	1.6	9.2	10.1	1.3
classic	Eden Vale	127	1.0	7.0	10.8	n/a
classic, low calorie	Eden Vale					
crunchy	Bodyline	61.0	1.4	6.0	3.7	n/a
fruity	Eden Vale	128	0.9	7.2	10.8	n/a
reduced calorie	Eden Vale	207	1.3	9.6	18.4	n/a
spicy	St Ivel Shape	93.0	1.9	4.8	7.5	1.8
	Eden Vale	201	1.4	12.5	16.5	n/a

with cheddar cheese	Boots	268	5.9	7.6	24.0	1.3
Coleslaw Dressing	Flora	Boots	63.0	0.2	2.6	5.8	n/a
	Kraft	449	2.0	24.0	39.0	n/a
Coley Fillet, steamed		99.0	23.3	nil	0.6	nil
Common Sense Oat Bran Flakes	Kellogg's	360	11.0	68.0	4.0	10.0
with raison & apple	Kellogg's	360	10.0	69.0	4.0	9.0
Complan, per serving original	Crookes Healthcare	247	11.4	32.0	8.0	n/a
banana	Crookes Healthcare	246	11.4	32.0	8.0	n/a
chicken	Crookes Healthcare	247	12.0	31.0	8.0	n/a
chocolate	Crookes Healthcare	246	11.4	32.0	8.0	n/a
mushroom	Crookes Healthcare	248	12.0	31.0	8.0	n/a
strawberry	Crookes Healthcare	246	11.4	32.0	8.0	n/a

All amounts given per 100g/100ml unless otherwise stated

Product	Brand	Calories kcal	Protein (g)	Carbo-hydrate (g)	Fat (g)	Dietary Fibre (g)
Compound Cooking Fat		894	Tr	Tr	99.3	nil
Condensed Milk						
sweetened, skimmed		267	10.0	60.0	0.2	nil
sweetened, whole		333	8.5	55.5	10.1	nil
Conservation Grade						
Porridge Oats	Jordans	396	13.5	71.9	8.9	6.3
Consomme	Crosse & Blackwell	20.0	4.0	0.9	Tr	Tr
condensed	Campbell's	13.0	2.3	0.9	nil	nil
Continental Meat						
Pizza, each	Birds Eye Gino Ginelli	750	36.0	102	25.0	n/a
Continental Mix	Ross	37.0	1.6	8.9	0.4	2.2
Contrast	Cadbury	490	4.9	61.9	26.6	n/a
Cook-In-Sauces (Homepride): see flavours						
Cook In The Pot Sauces & Mixes (Crosse & Blackwell): see flavours						
Cookeen Cooking fat	Van Den Berghs	900	nil	nil	100	nil

Cookies	Cadbury's	467	6.1	68.6	20.6	n/a
Cooking Mixes & Sauces (Colman's): see flavours						
Coolmints, each	Trebor Bassett	4.0	n/a	1.5	Tr	n/a
Coq au Vin	Baxters	77.0	10.5	3.2	2.6	0.4
Coq au Vin Casserole Mix, as sold	Colman's	299	7.7	n/a	1.5	n/a
Coq au Vin Cook-In-Sauce	Homepride	48.0	0.5	7.6	n/a	n/a
Cook-In-Sauce Classic	Homepride	47.0	0.8	10.3	n/a	n/a
Coriander & Herb Flavoured Rice	Batchelors	370	8.4	77.1	5.3	n/a
Corn Cobs, frozen	Green Giant	100	n/a	n/a	1.0	n/a
Corn Flakes	Kellogg's	380	8.0	84.0	0.7	1.0
	Sunblest	390	7.6	86.9	1.0	2.6
frosted	Sunblest	390	5.6	88.1	1.4	1.2
high fibre	Ryvita	370	8.3	80.9	1.3	9.3
Corn Oil	Mazola	900	Tr	nil	99.9	n/a
Corn on the Cob, whole, raw		54.0	2.0	9.9	1.0	0.9

All amounts given per 100g/100ml unless otherwise stated

Product	Brand	Calories kcal	Protein (g)	Carbo-hydrate (g)	Fat (g)	Dietary Fibre (g)
boiled						
frozen	Findus	66.0	2.5	11.6	1.4	1.3
frozen, premium choice	Ross	124	4.1	21.6	2.4	3.7
		101	3.1	22.7	1.0	2.7
Corned Beef, canned		217	26.9	nil	26.9	nil
Corned Beef Hash	Fray Bentos	111	6.6	11.8	4.4	n/a
Cornetto (Wall's): *see flavours*						
Cornflour		354	0.6	92.0	0.7	0.1
Cornish Dairy Ice Cream	Lyons Maid	92.0	1.9	11.3	4.4	n/a
Cornish Pastie	Ross	332	8.0	31.1	20.4	0.9
Hungryman Giant		258	7.3	23.9	15.2	1.0
Cornish King Cone	Lyons Maid	221	3.4	24.6	12.2	n/a
Cornish Strawberry King Cone	Lyons Maid	155	2.1	18.2	8.7	n/a
Cornish Wafers	Jacob's	506	7.6	54.6	30.1	2.3
***Cottage Cheese** (see also flavours)* plain		98.0	13.8	2.1	3.9	nil

with additions						
reduced fat						
diet	Eden Vale Bodyline	95.0	12.8	2.6	3.8	Tr
	St Ivel Shape	78.0	13.3	3.3	1.4	Tr
Cough Candy Twists, each	Trebor Bassett	26.0	n/a	7.0	n/a	n/a
Country Beef Cook-In-Sauce	Homepride	37.0	0.8	7.3	n/a	n/a
Country Beef Recipe Sauce, dry, as sold	Knorr	319	9.6	58.0	7.0	4.2
Country Chicken Recipe Sauce, dry, as sold	Knorr	352	4.4	58.4	12.8	3.8
Country Crisp with Strawberries	Jordans	392	7.4	57.2	16.4	5.4
Country Crunch Biscuits	Peek Frean	445	7.8	67.6	17.8	3.6
Country Delight Soya Desserts (Granose): see flavours						
Country Garden Soup	Baxters	28.0	0.7	5.4	0.5	0.8
Country Grain Multigrain Wholemeal Bread	Hovis	218	9.5	37.1	2.9	7.1

All amounts given per 100g/100ml unless otherwise stated

Product	Brand	Calories kcal	Protein (g)	Carbo-hydrate (g)	Fat (g)	Dietary Fibre (g)
Country Mix Vegetables	Findus	55.0	2.4	10.6	0.4	4.6
	Ross	30.0	2.3	7.6	0.3	3.0
Country Sausage Cook-In-Sauce	Homepride	37.0	1.1	6.7	n/a	n/a
Country Slices, each	Mr Kipling	120	1.4	18.6	5.0	n/a
Country Stir Fry Vegetables (fried), 28g/1oz	Birds Eye	12.0	0.5	1.5	0.5	n/a
Country Store	Kellogg's	350	9.0	69.0	4.0	6.0
Country Style Chicken Casserole Recipe Sauce	Knorr	34.0	0.8	8.0	0.1	n/a
Country Vegetable & Beef Soup	Heinz Weight Watchers	22.0	1.3	3.7	0.3	0.7
Country Vegetable Soup, low calorie	Heinz Weight Watchers	22.0	0.9	3.8	0.3	1.1
Courgettes (zucchini, squash), raw boiled		18.0	1.8	1.8	0.4	0.9
		19.0	2.0	2.0	0.4	1.2

fried in corn oil		63.0	2.6	2.6	4.8	1.2
Crab, boiled						
canned		127	20.1	nil	5.2	nil
		81.0	18.1	nil	0.9	nil
Crabmeat in Brine	Armour	80.0	16.0	nil	nil	nil
Crab Paste	Shippams	167	n/a	n/a	n/a	n/a
Cracker Barrel Cheddar						
Cheese	Kraft	406	26.0	nil	34.0	n/a
Crackerbread, per slice	Ryvita	20.0	0.6	3.8	0.2	0.1
high fibre, per slice	Ryvita	14.0	0.6	2.6	0.1	0.6
Cranberry Jelly	Baxters	255	Tr	68.0	Tr	1.7
Cranberry Sauce	Baxters	126	0.1	33.3	nil	1.4
	Burgess	205	nil	50.7	nil	1.2
Cream, fresh (pasteurised)						
clotted		586	1.6	2.3	63.5	nil
double		449	1.7	2.7	48.0	nil
half		148	3.0	4.3	13.3	nil
single		198	2.6	4.1	19.1	nil

All amounts given per 100g/100ml unless otherwise stated

Product	Brand	Calories kcal	Protein (g)	Carbo-hydrate (g)	Fat (g)	Dietary Fibre (g)
soured		205	2.9	3.8	19.9	nil
whipping		373	2.0	3.1	39.3	nil
Cream, imitation						
Dessert Top	Nestlé	291	2.4	6.0	28.8	Tr
Dream Topping						
made with whole milk	Bird's	182	3.8	12.1	13.5	Tr
made with semi-skimmed	Bird's	166	3.9	12.2	11.7	Tr
Elmlea, single	Van Den Berghs	190	3.2	4.1	18.0	0.3
Elmlea, double	Van Den Berghs	454	2.5	3.2	48.0	0.1
Elmlea, whipping	Van Den Berghs	319	2.5	3.2	33.0	0.1
Tip top	Nestlé	110	5.0	8.5	6.5	Tr
Cream, sterilised, canned		239	2.5	3.7	23.9	nil
Cream, UHT, aerosol spray		309	1.9	3.5	32.0	nil
Cream Cheese		439	3.1	Tr	47.4	nil
Cream Crackers	Jacob's	440	9.5	68.3	16.3	2.2
		418	8.5	67.6	14.5	2.8
Cream of Asparagus Soup	Baxters	66.0	0.9	4.8	4.9	0.2

128

condensed	Heinz	44.0	0.8	4.4	2.6	0.1
	Campbell's	87.0	1.4	8.0	5.5	0.4
Cream of Celery Soup condensed	Heinz	44.0	0.9	3.5	2.9	0.4
	Campbell's	93.0	1.3	6.2	7.0	0.6
Cream of Chicken Soup, canned, ready to serve		58.0	1.7	4.5	3.8	N
condensed, ready to serve		98.0	2.6	6.0	7.2	N
Cream of Cornish Ice Cream	Wall's	90.0	2.0	12.0	3.0	n/a
Cream of Courgette Soup	Baxters	54.0	1.0	5.5	3.2	0.7
Cream of Leek Soup	Baxters	45.0	0.6	5.8	2.4	0.4
Cream of Mushroom Soup, canned, ready to serve		53	1.1	3.9	3.8	N
condensed	Campbell's	98.0	1.3	6.9	7.2	0.3
Cream of Pheasant soup	Baxters	60.0	2.0	4.9	3.6	0.2
Cream of Prawn Soup, condensed	Campbell's	108	2.4	8.4	7.2	0.1
Cream of Scampi Soup	Baxters	54.0	2.2	5.6	2.7	0.1

All amounts given per 100g/100ml unless otherwise stated

Product	Brand	Calories kcal	Protein (g)	Carbohydrate (g)	Fat (g)	Dietary Fibre (g)
Cream of Smoked Salmon Soup, condensed	Campbell's	123	5.6	7.6	7.9	0.1
Cream of Smoked Scotch Salmon Soup	Baxters	95.0	4.2	5.7	6.1	0.1
Cream of Tomato Soup						
canned, ready to serve		55.0	0.8	5.9	3.3	N
condensed, ready to serve		123	1.7	14.6	6.8	N
Cream Soda	Barr	29.0	n/a	n/a	n/a	n/a
	Corona	26.0	n/a	7.0	n/a	n/a
traditional style	Idris	20.0	n/a	5.2	n/a	n/a
Cream Style Corn	Green Giant	77.0	n/a	n/a	nil	n/a
Creamed Horseradish	Ambrosia	192	2.9	14.6	10.0	n/a
Creamed Macaroni	Ambrosia	92.0	4.0	14.6	1.9	n/a
Creamed Rice	Ambrosia	91.0	3.4	15.2	1.8	n/a
	Libby	88.0	3.2	15.2	1.6	0.2
low fat	Ambrosia	75.0	3.5	13.2	0.9	0.2

Creamed Sago	Ambrosia	82.0	2.9	13.2	1.8	n/a
Creamed Semolina	Ambrosia	84.0	3.6	13.2	1.9	n/a
Creamed Smatana	Raines	130	4.7	5.6	10.0	nil
Creamed Spinach	Findus	58.0	3.1	4.3	3.2	0.5
Creamed Tapioca	Ambrosia	83.0	2.9	13.8	1.8	n/a
Creamed Tomato Soup	Crosse & Blackwell	76.0	0.7	10.0	3.7	0.1
Creamed Tomatoes	Napolina	12.0	0.7	3.3	Tr	0.7
Creamy Chicken & Broccoli Bake, per pack	Birds Eye	56.0	1.1	7.2	2.7	1.1
	MenuMaster	235	18.0	15.0	12.0	n/a
Creamy Highland Veg Soup	Baxters	56.0	1.1	7.2	2.7	1.1
Creme Caramel		109	3.0	20.6	2.2	N
	Eden Vale	139	3.8	21.0	5.0	n/a
	St Ivel	110	3.8	21.1	1.7	n/a
Creme De Creme Ice Cream Cups (Lyons Maid): see flavours						
Creme Eggs		385	4.1	58.0	16.8	Tr

All amounts given per 100g/100ml unless otherwise stated

Product	Brand	Calories kcal	Protein (g)	Carbohydrate (g)	Fat (g)	Dietary Fibre (g)
Crinkle Cut Chips: _see Chips_						
Crisp 'n' Dry, solid/oil	Van Den Berghs	900	nil	nil	100	n/a
Crispbread Lunchpacks						
with low fat dairy spread with low fat cheese	Boots Shapers	432	26.5	57.9	10.5	2.1
& mushroom dairy spread with reduced calorie	Boots Shapers	436	26.5	58.5	10.7	2.1
Brussels pate	Boots Shapers	449	27.5	55.6	10.5	2.7
Crisps: _see flavours_						
Crispy Chinese with Quorn Stir Fry	Ross	65.0	4.9	10.6	1.0	1.6
Crispy Cod, Haddock, etc: _see Cod, Haddock, etc_						
Crispy Muesli	Jordans	352	10.4	63.7	6.2	8.5
Crispy Toffee Cake	California Cake & Cookie Co.	462	5.9	69.8	35.4	n/a
Crispy Topped Shepherds	Batchelors					

Pie	Microchef Meal	134	6.8	11.1	7.2	n/a
Croissants						
Croquette Potatoes, baked	Birds Eye	360	8.3	38.3	20.3	2.5
Crostinos, grilled, each	Findus	110	5.0	9.0	1.0	n/a
Crumble Mix, as sold	Whitworths	466	5.5	68.4	20.8	0.2
Crumpet Fingers	Mothers Pride	185	6.2	37.1	0.8	1.9
Crumpets	Mothers Pride	185	6.2	37.1	0.8	1.9
	Sunblest	182	5.7	37.9	1.0	1.4
Crunch & Fudge Cool Top Mix, made up, per serving	Homepride	204	2.0	28.0	9.0	n/a
Crunch 'n' Slim (Crookes Healthcare); *see flavours*						
Crunch Creams	Peek Frean	477	5.1	66.5	23.0	1.9
Crunch Mixes: *see flavours*						
Crunchie, per bar	Cadbury	195	1.9	30.5	8.0	n/a
Crunchy Bemax: *see Bemax*						

All amounts given per 100g/100ml unless otherwise stated

Product	Brand	Calories kcal	Protein (g)	Carbo-hydrate (g)	Fat (g)	Dietary Fibre (g)
Crunchy Cheese Wotsits, per pack	Golden Wonder	196	2.4	18.9	12.3	n/a
Crunchy Nut Cereal	Granose	493	10.5	59.3	23.8	n/a
Crunchy Nut Cornflakes	Kellogg's	400	7.0	83.0	4.0	1.0
Crusha (Burgess): see flavours						
Crusty Cobs, each	Sunblest	162	5.7	29.4	2.3	1.1
Crusty Ploughmans Rolls	Mothers Pride	289	10.3	51.9	3.6	n/a
Cube Sugar, white	Tate & Lyle	398	nil	99.9	nil	nil
Cucumber, raw		10.0	0.7	1.5	0.1	0.6
Cucumber & Green Pepper Chutney	Baxters	85.0	0.5	22.1	0.1	1.4
Cucumber Sandwich Spread	Heinz	187	1.3	19.6	11.5	0.7
Cullen Skink Soup	Baxters	85.0	6.6	7.9	3.2	0.5
Cultured Buttermilk	Raines	40.0	4.3	5.5	0.1	nil
Cup Cakes, chocolate	Lyons	338	2.2	77.0	4.2	0.5

assorted	Lyons	353	2.1	78.6	5.5	0.4
Curacao		311	Tr	28.3	nil	nil
Curly Kale, raw boiled		33.0 / 24.0	3.4 / 2.4	1.4 / 1.0	1.6 / 1.1	3.1 / 2.8
Curly Wurly, per bar	Cadbury	130	1.5	20.1	5.2	n/a
Currant Buns		296	7.6	52.7	7.5	N
Currants, dried		267	2.3	67.8	0.4	1.9
Curried Beans with Sultanas	Heinz	117	5.3	20.7	1.4	6.4
Curried Beef & Vegetables	Tyne Brand	87.0	3.7	11.0	3.4	n/a
Curried Chicken Toast Topper	Heinz	78.0	7.7	7.3	2.0	0.3
Curried Chicken with Rice Soup	Heinz	52.0	1.4	6.2	2.4	0.2
Curried Fruit Chutney	Sharwood	153	0.6	38.1	0.2	1.0
Curried Vegetables with Coriander Soup	Heinz	39.0	1.1	7.5	0.5	1.1
Curry Casserole Recipe Sauce	Knorr	91.0	1.4	13.4	3.9	n/a
Curry Cook-In-Sauce	Homepride	111	0.8	8.8	n/a	n/a

All amounts given per 100g/100ml unless otherwise stated

Product	Brand	Calories kcal	Protein (g)	Carbohydrate (g)	Fat (g)	Dietary Fibre (g)
Curry Dip, per pack	Kavli	350	6.9	6.0	33.3	n/a
Curry Sauce	HP	137	1.6	24.0	3.8	n/a
canned	Sharwood	228	1.0	44.3	0.5	1.9
		78.0	1.5	7.1	5.0	N
Custard						
made up with whole milk		117	3.7	16.6	4.5	Tr
made up with skimmed milk		79.0	3.8	16.8	0.1	Tr
canned		95.0	2.6	15.4	3.0	0.1
canned, low fat	Ambrosia	75.0	3.0	12.5	1.4	nil
Custard Creams	Crawfords	513	5.5	67.6	24.2	1.5
	Peek Frean	483	5.3	71.7	21.2	1.3
diabetic	Boots	467	6.7	65.0	20.0	20.
Custard Tarts		277	6.3	32.4	14.5	1.2

D

Dairy Box	Rowntree Mackintosh	447	5.0	67.1	19.5	n/a
Dairy Cream Eclairs, each	Birds Eye	145	2.5	10.0	11.0	n/a
Dairy Creme Vienna Dessert						
chocolate	Chambourcy	149	3.6	20.7	5.7	0.3
strawberry	Chambourcy	134	3.4	19.4	4.8	0.3
Dairy Crunch, milk	Rowntree Mackintosh	500	8.0	60.0	27.0	n/a
white	Rowntree Mackintosh	530	8.0	60.0	30.0	n/a
mini bars	Rowntree Mackintosh	492	7.1	66.0	24.0	n/a
Dairy Fudge, each	Trebor Bassett	43.0	Tr	6.8	1.9	n/a

All amounts given per 100g/100ml unless otherwise stated

Product	Brand	Calories kcal	Protein (g)	Carbohydrate (g)	Fat (g)	Dietary Fibre (g)
Dairy Ice Cream: see Ice Cream						
Dairy Milk Chocolate	Cadbury	520	7.7	58.7	29.9	n/a
Dairylea Cheese Food Slices	Kraft	315	18.0	5.0	25.0	n/a
Dairylea Cheese Spread	Kraft	282	13.0	6.0	23.0	n/a
with bacon	Kraft	280	12.0	6.5	23.0	n/a
with onion	Kraft	275	10.5	6.5	23.0	n/a
Dairylea Light Cheese & Skimmed Milk Spread	Kraft	185	16.0	6.0	11.0	n/a
Dairy Slices, low fat, each	Delight	36.0	3.0	0.6	2.4	n/a
Dairy/Fat Spread (see also brands & flavours)		662	0.4	Tr	73.4	nil
Dairy Toffees, each	Trebor Bassett	31.0	Tr	4.5	1.4	n/a
Damsons						
raw (weighed with stones)		34.0	0.5	8.6	Tr	1.6
stewed with sugar		107	1.3	26.9	0.1	1.5
Dandelion & Burdock	Barr	28.0	n/a	n/a	n/a	n/a
	Corona	20.0	n/a	5.2	n/a	n/a
low calorie	Barr	1.5	n/a	n/a	n/a	n/a

138

		28.0	n/a	7.5	n/a	n/a
traditional style	Idris	347	20.1	Tr	29.6	nil
Danish Brie with Chives	St Ivel	448	13.0	Tr	44.0	n/a
Danish Pastries		374	5.8	51.3	17.6	1.6
Danish Toaster Bread	Mothers Pride	246	8.3	46.5	2.2	3.6
	Sunblest	235	7.6	45.7	2.4	2.3
Danish White Bread	Mothers Pride	246	8.3	46.5	2.2	3.6
	Sunblest	235	7.6	45.7	2.4	2.3
Dansak Classic Curry Sauce	Homepride	96.0	3.0	12.9	n/a	n/a
Dark & Aromatic Chinese Sauce Mix, as sold	Sharwood	271	3.0	67.0	0.9	n/a
Dark & Golden Choc Ice, each	Wall's	124	1.3	11.5	8.5	n/a
Dark Brown Soft Sugar	Tate & Lyle	380	0.2	95.0	nil	nil
Date & Walnut Wholemeal Cake Mix	Granose	402	11.4	55.9	11.0	2.0
Date Bar, each	Granose	87.5	0.7	18.7	1.0	2.0
Dates, raw, weighed with stones		227	2.8	57.1	0.2	1.5

All amounts given per 100g/100ml unless otherwise stated

Product	Brand	Calories kcal	Protein (g)	Carbohydrate (g)	Fat (g)	Dietary Fibre (g)
dried						
block	Whitworths	268	2.3	68.1	0.4	3.4
stoned	Whitworths	256	2.1	66.0	Tr	9.0
		274	2.2	70.7	Tr	9.4
Deep Crust Pizza Mix, as sold	Homepride Perfect	247	10.0	50.0	3.0	n/a
Deep Dish Lasagne Verdi	Findus Dinner Supreme	144	9.0	10.5	7.1	1.0
Delicately Flavoured Rice (Batchelors): *see flavours*						
Delight Cream Alternative						
single	Van Den Berghs	18.0	0.5	1.0	1.4	n/a
double	Van Den Berghs	36.0	0.4	0.6	3.6	n/a
Delight Low Fat Spread	Van Den Berghs	376	4.4	1.3	39.2	n/a
extra low	Van Den Berghs	226	3.0	9.0	20.0	n/a
Delight Pates (Van Den Berghs): *see flavours*						
Delights	Rowntree Mackintosh	391	4.3	65.2	14.4	n/a

Deluxe Muesli	Boots	349	9.0	57.0	11.0	9.5
Demerara Sugar		394	0.5	104.5	nil	nil
Derby Cheese		402	24.2	0.1	33.9	nil
Derby Scones	Mothers Pride	385	6.4	55.0	15.1	nil
Desert Gold Cider	HP Bulmer	53.0	n/a	n/a	n/a	n/a
Desiccated Coconut: *see Coconut*						
Dessert Mixes (Dietade): *see flavours*						
Dessert Pies, apple	Lyons	349	3.0	57.1	13.6	1.5
Dessert White Sauce	Ambrosia	98.0	2.9	14.6	3.1	n/a
Devon Custard	Ambrosia	102	2.8	15.8	3.1	n/a
Devon Sponge Cake Mix, as sold	Green's	368	2.0	32.0	11.0	n/a
Devonshire Cheesecake						
blackcurrant	St Ivel	250	6.3	26.5	14.0	n/a
lemon & sultana	St Ivel	276	6.7	29.8	15.2	n/a
strawberry	St Ivel	250	6.3	26.5	14.0	n/a

All amounts given per 100g/100ml unless otherwise stated

Product	Brand	Calories kcal	Protein (g)	Carbo-hydrate (g)	Fat (g)	Dietary Fibre (g)
Dhansak Curry Sauce, canned	Sharwood	92.0	2.8	9.7	4.6	1.8
Diabetic Products (Boots, Dietade): *see flavours*						
Diet Drinks: *see flavours*						
Diet Ski Yogurt (Eden Vale): *see flavours*						
Dietade (Applefords): *see products*						
Digestive Biscuits						
chocolate		493	6.8	66.5	24.1	2.2
plain		471	6.3	68.6	20.9	2.2
Dijon Mustard	Colman's	178	9.0	n/a	12.0	n/a
Dinner Balls	Granose	145	12.0	8.0	7.0	0.1
Dinner Supreme (Findus); *see flavours*						
Disney Pasta						
fun pasta	Crosse & Blackwell	60.0	1.6	12.5	0.3	0.1
fun pasta tomato soup	Crosse &					

142

	Brand					
mini ravioli	Blackwell Crosse & Blackwell	70.0	1.1	10.1	2.9	0.1
pasta bolognese	Blackwell Crosse & Blackwell	75.0	1.6	12.4	2.0	0.4
pasta & sausages	Blackwell Crosse & Blackwell	70.0	3.0	10.7	1.6	0.4
pasta with beans	Blackwell Crosse & Blackwell	95.0	3.4	10.1	4.8	0.2
	Blackwell Crosse & Blackwell	80.0	3.4	15.8	0.5	3.4
Ditto	Tunnock's	457	4.3	65.8	22.8	n/a
Dolmio Pasta & Pasta Sauces: see flavours						
Dopiaza Classic Curry Sauce	Homepride	76.0	1.3	10.7	n/a	n/a
Double Cheese Pizza Slice	McCain Pizza Pantry	219	10.8	28.0	7.9	n/a
Double Choc Chip Cookies	Huntley & Palmer	473	5.8	61.7	24.2	1.5
Double Chocolate Chip Cookie	California Cake & Cookie Co.	448	5.2	56.4	24.0	0.9

All amounts given per 100g/100ml unless otherwise stated

Product	Brand	Calories kcal	Protein (g)	Carbo-hydrate (g)	Fat (g)	Dietary Fibre (g)
Double Decker, per bar	Cadbury	235	3.1	34.3	10.4	n/a
Double Gloucester Cheese		405	24.6	0.1	34.0	nil
Double Gloucester with Chives & Onion	St Ivel	400	24.3	1.0	33.4	n/a
Doublemint Chewing gum	Wrigley	306	nil	2.4	nil	nil
Doughnuts, jam ring		336	5.7	48.8	14.5	N
		397	6.1	47.2	21.7	N
Dream Choc Bars, each original	Wall's	200	3.0	20.0	13.0	n/a
fruit & nut	Wall's	215	3.0	22.0	13.0	n/a
Dream Topping (Bird's): *see Cream, imitation*						
Dressed Crab	Young's	132	17.2	4.4	5.1	Tr
Dried Fruit Mix	Whitworths	287	2.5	72.2	Tr	4.0
Dried Milk (see also brands) skimmed, as sold		348	36.1	52.9	0.6	nil
Drifter	Rowntree					

144

	Mackintosh	469	4.5	68.8	21.4	n/a
Drinking Chocolate, powder		366	5.5	77.4	6.0	N
made up with whole milk		90.0	3.4	10.6	4.1	Tr
made up with semi-skimmed milk		71.0	3.5	10.8	1.9	Tr
Dripping, beef		891	Tr	Tr	99.0	nil
Dry Ginger Ale	Schweppes	15.0	n/a	4.0	n/a	n/a
Dry Roasted Nuts, per pack	Golden Wonder	278	13.3	15.7	18.5	n/a
Duck						
meat only, roast		189	25.3	nil	9.7	nil
meat, fat & skin, roast		339	19.6	nil	29.0	nil
Dumplings		208	2.8	24.5	11.7	0.9
Dutch Apple Tart	McVitie's	232	3.4	34.7	9.2	0.9
Dutch Cheese: *see Edam, Gouda*						
Dutch Pea Soup	Rakusen	23.0	2.0	4.5	0.5	n/a
Dutch Shortcake Biscuits	Huntley & Palmer	505	7.0	55.0	29.0	n/a

All amounts given per 100g/100ml unless otherwise stated

E

Product	Brand	Calories kcal	Protein (g)	Carbo-hydrate (g)	Fat (g)	Dietary Fibre (g)
Easy Cook White Rice, boiled		138	2.6	30.9	1.3	0.1
Eccles Cakes		475	3.9	59.3	26.4	1.6
Echo Margarine	Van Den Berghs	732	0.1	0.4	81.0	n/a
Eclairs, frozen dairy cream	Birds Eye	396	5.6	26.1	30.6	0.8
		145	2.5	10.0	11.0	n/a
Economy Burgers, each	Birds Eye Steakhouse	90.0	8.0	3.5	5.0	n/a
Edam Cheese		333	26.0	Tr	25.4	nil
Egg Custard Mix, made up, per serving	Homepride Perfect	148	5.5	17.5	6.0	n/a
Egg Free Dressing	Flora	72.0	Tr	1.1	8.0	n/a

		208	4.2	25.7	10.6	0.4
Egg Fried Rice						
Eggplant: see Aubergine						
Eggs, chicken						
raw, whole		147	12.5	Tr	10.8	nil
raw, white only		36.0	9.0	Tr	Tr	nil
raw, yolk only		339	16.1	Tr	30.5	nil
boiled		147	12.5	Tr	10.8	nil
fried		179	13.6	Tr	13.9	nil
poached		147	12.5	Tr	10.8	nil
scrambled with milk		247	10.7	0.6	22.6	nil
Eggs, duck						
raw, whole		163	14.3	Tr	11.8	nil
8 Fruit Muesli	Granose	408	10.5	62.8	14.4	n/a
Elmlea Cream Alternative: see Cream, imitation						
English Butter Garnish						
for garnish	Dairy Crest	696	0.5	1.8	76.0	nil
garlic	Dairy Crest	706	0.5	0.5	78.0	nil
mixed herb	Dairy Crest	682	0.5	0.5	80.0	nil

All amounts given per 100g/100ml unless otherwise stated

Product	Brand	Calories kcal	Protein (g)	Carbo-hydrate (g)	Fat (g)	Dietary Fibre (g)
parsley & lemon	Dairy Crest	715	0.5	0.5	79.0	nil
English Cheddar Cheese		412	25.5	0.1	34.4	nil
English Farmhouse Vegetable Soup	Campbell's	29.0	1.2	5.65	0.1	1.9
English Mustard	Burgess	179	7.9	19.5	7.2	0.2
	Colman's	184	7.0	n/a	9.3	n/a
English Supreme Chicken Soup	Campbell's	80.0	1.9	4.5	6.0	0.1
English Supreme Soup mushroom	Campbell's	83.0	1.0	7.1	5.7	0.2
tomato	Campbell's	108	0.9	9.7	7.3	nil
Evaporated Milk, whole	Carnation	151	8.4	8.5	9.4	nil
full cream	Nestlé Ideal	160	8.2	11.5	9.0	n/a
		160	8.2	11.5	9.0	n/a
Everton Mints, each	Trebor Bassett	23.0	n/a	5.9	0.08	n/a
Exotic Fresh Fruit Salad,						

per pack	Boots Shapers	46.0	n/a	n/a	n/a	n/a
Exotic Juice	St Ivel Real	39.0	0.2	10.0	0.1	n/a
Extra Chunky Vegetables Pasta Sauce	Dolmio	35.0	1.9	6.9	Tr	n/a
Extra Garlic Pasta Sauce	Dolmio	38.0	1.1	7.3	0.5	n/a
Extra Herbs Pasta Sauce	Dolmio	26.0	1.0	5.5	Tr	n/a
Extra Strong Mints, roll, each	Trebor Bassett	10.0	n/a	2.6	n/a	n/a

Fab, each	Lyons Maid	85.0	0.5	15.0	3.0	n/a
Faggots	Ross	268	11.1	15.3	18.5	N
	Mr Brain's	189	6.6	11.8	13.0	0.5
in rich sauce		143	7.0	13.0	7.0	n/a

All amounts given per 100g/100ml unless otherwise stated

Product	Brand	Calories kcal	Protein (g)	Carbohydrate (g)	Fat (g)	Dietary Fibre (g)
Faggots in Tomato & Onion Sauce	Mr Brain's	132	6.9	10.3	5.3	n/a
Faggots, Jacket Potatoes, Peas & Sauce	Mr Brain's	82.0	5.0	7.5	3.7	n/a
Family Soft Wholemeal Bread	Allinson	220	10.8	37.0	3.4	6.5
Family Wheatgerm Bread	Hovis	228	9.7	39.5	2.9	4.5
Fancies, chocolate	Lyons	488	5.3	52.6	29.9	0.3
Fancy Iced Cakes		407	3.8	68.8	14.9	N
Farmhouse Baps, each	Sunblest	113	3.9	24.1	2.3	0.9
Farmhouse Biscuits	Jacob's	415	8.2	59.9	17.6	4.5
Farmhouse Chicken Casserole with Veg & Rice	Findus Lean Cuisine	80.0	5.3	11.4	1.4	1.5
Farmhouse Soups (Heinz): *see flavours*						
Farmhouse Vegetable Hotpot Casserole Mix, as sold	Colman's	313	6.2	n/a	3.9	n/a

Farrow Peas, canned	Batchelors	80.0	6.2	13.7	0.4	n/a
Fast Cook Recipe Meals (Ross): see flavours						
Feast, each	Wall's	290	3.5	21.0	22.0	n/a
mint	Wall's	280	6.7	20.0	21.0	n/a
Fennel, Florence, raw		12.0	0.9	1.8	0.2	2.4
boiled		11.0	0.9	1.5	0.2	2.3
Feta Cheese		250	15.6	1.5	20.2	nil
55 Juice						
apple	Britvic	45.0	n/a	11.9	n/a	n/a
grapefruit	Britvic	50.0	n/a	13.3	n/a	n/a
orange	Britvic	52.0	n/a	13.8	n/a	n/a
pineapple	Britvic	51.0	n/a	13.6	n/a	n/a
Fig Fruit Snack Bar	Granose	80.0	1.0	16.7	1.0	2.5
Fig Rolls	Crawfords	405	3.4	67.9	11.4	2.5
	Jacob's	340	3.9	67.4	6.9	5.7
Figaro Choc Ice	Lyons Maid	275	3.4	24.9	18.1	n/a
dark	Lyons Maid	246	3.1	24.4	17.5	n/a

All amounts given per 100g/100ml unless otherwise stated

Product	Brand	Calories kcal	Protein (g)	Carbohydrate (g)	Fat (g)	Dietary Fibre (g)
Figs, dried						
ready to eat		209	3.3	48.6	1.5	7.5
		122	0.4	7.2	Tr	6.9
Figs in Syrup	Libby	88.0	n/a	n/a	Tr	n/a
Filet-o-Fish, each	McDonald's	332	17.6	41.6	11.7	3.0
Finger Biscuits, milk	Cadbury	509	7.1	68.8	24.7	n/a
Finger Rolls, each	Sunblest	102	3.5	17.6	1.4	0.6
Finger Shortbread	McVitie's	525	6.1	63.1	27.1	2.0
Fish & Chips	Ross Chip Shop	175	5.9	18.8	8.8	0.7
Fish 'n' Chips Candy, each	Trebor Bassett	34.0	n/a	3.2	1.8	n/a
Fish & Potato Bake	Ross Recipe Meal	90.0	5.8	8.1	3.9	0.3
Fish & Tomato Gratin	Ross Recipe Meal	121	7.3	9.3	6.2	0.4
Fish Cakes (see also flavours)						
fried		188	9.1	15.1	10.5	N
battered	Ross Chip Shop	120	9.2	19.7	0.8	0.8
	Ross Chip Shop	194	8.1	16.5	10.9	0.6

value, each	Birds Eye	85.0	4.5	9.0	3.5	n/a
Fish Cubes	Knorr	296	18.9	9.5	20.5	0.9
Fish, Cheese & Onion Scrunchy	Findus	247	6.8	21.2	15.0	1.2
Fish Feast						
in cheese sauce, each	Birds Eye	220	12.0	19.0	11.0	n/a
in garlic butter, each	Birds Eye	195	12.0	17.0	9.5	n/a
Fish Fillets, skinless	Ross Chip Shop	230	10.5	14.3	14.7	0.5
Fish fingers (see also flavours)						
fried in oil		233	13.5	17.2	12.7	0.6
grilled	Ross	214	15.1	19.3	9.0	0.7
		179	11.4	16.8	8.1	0.7
each	Birds Eye	45.0	3.0	2.0	4.0	n/a
prime, each	Birds Eye	45.0	3.0	2.0	4.0	n/a
Fish Paste		169	15.3	3.7	10.4	0.2
Fish Pie		102	8.0	12.3	3.0	0.7
Fish Portions	Ross Chip Shop	225	11.3	12.7	14.5	0.5
in crispy crumb	Ross	186	11.0	13.9	9.9	0.6

All amounts given per 100g/100ml unless otherwise stated

Product	Brand	Calories kcal	Protein (g)	Carbo-hydrate (g)	Fat (g)	Dietary Fibre (g)
Fish Shop Fish (Ross): *see flavours*						
Fish Steaks						
in butter sauce	Ross	93.0	9.4	2.9	4.9	0.1
in parsley sauce	Ross	90.0	10.2	2.9	4.2	0.1
Fish with Tomato & Basil Pasta Sauce, dry, as sold	Buitoni	395	12.7	53.5	14.5	1.4
Fisherman's Pie, per pack	Birds Eye MenuMaster	375	27.0	26.0	19.0	n/a
Fisherman's Pie with Broccoli & Sweetcorn	Findus Lean Cuisine	83.0	7.0	10.0	1.7	0.9
Fisherman's Pottage	Baxters	41.0	3.7	3.3	1.6	0.1
Five Centres, per bar	Cadbury	210	1.7	36.8	7.4	n/a
Five Fruits Drink	Del Monte Fruit Burst	46.0	0.2	11.1	Tr	n/a
Fivepints Milk Powder, made up, per pint	St Ivel	260	12.5	25.9	13.6	n/a

Flageolet Beans	Batchelors	96.0	7.3	15.8	0.8	n/a
Flake, each	Cadbury	170	2.8	19.9	9.7	n/a
Flake Cakes, all flavours, each	Cadbury	99.0	1.6	13.0	4.9	n/a
Flake Ice Cream	Wall's Dream	148	3.2	17.0	8.0	n/a
Flaky Pastry: see Pastry						
Flan	Lyons	346	6.4	67.0	7.6	1.2
Flapjack Slice	Peek Frean	491	5.5	61.3	26.1	2.9
Flapjacks		484	4.5	60.4	26.6	2.7
Flintstones in Tomato Sauce	Heinz	62.0	1.8	13.0	0.3	0.6
Flora						
baking	Van Den Berghs	736	nil	nil	82.0	n/a
cooking fat, white	Van Den Berghs	900	nil	nil	100	n/a
margarine	Van Den Berghs	728	0.2	1.3	80.0	n/a
margarine, extra light	Van Den Berghs	373	4.3	0.4	39.0	n/a
sunflower oil	Van Den Berghs	900	nil	nil	100	n/a
Flora Cream Alternative single	Van Den Berghs	30.0	0.5	0.7	2.8	n/a

All amounts given per 100g/100ml unless otherwise stated

Product	Brand	Calories kcal	Protein (g)	Carbohydrate (g)	Fat (g)	Dietary Fibre (g)
double	Van Den Berghs	69.0	0.4	0.5	7.3	n/a
Florida Orange Mini Juice, each	Wall's	25.0	Tr	7.0	Tr	n/a
Florida Salad	St Ivel Shape	126	0.4	10.9	9.3	n/a
Florida Sponge	Mr Kipling	321	3.5	60.7	8.7	n/a
Florida Wafer	Tunnock's	519	5.1	64.0	29.0	n/a
Flour, wheat						
brown		323	12.6	68.5	1.8	6.4
white, breadmaking		341	11.5	75.3	1.4	3.1
white, plain		341	9.4	77.7	1.3	3.1
white, self-raising		330	8.9	75.6	1.2	3.1
wholemeal		310	12.7	63.9	2.2	9.0
Folies	Huntley & Palmer	468	4.5	71.1	18.5	n/a
Folies au Chocolat	Huntley & Palmer	500	4.2	62.3	26.1	n/a

Forest Fruit Fromage Frais	Ski	140	6.7	14.5	6.5	n/a
Forest Fruit Juice Drink (carton)	Ribena	52.0	Tr	13.9	n/a	n/a
Forest Fruits Yogurt						
low calorie	Gold Ski	108	5.3	16.3	2.8	n/a
low calorie, French style	St Ivel Shape	41.0	4.7	5.6	0.1	n/a
	St Ivel Shape	40.0	4.8	5.3	0.1	n/a
Forest Fruits Yogurt Mousse Slice	Boots Shapers	162	3.6	23.0	6.8	1.0
Foresta Pasta Sauce	Dolmio	131	1.1	4.6	12.0	n/a
Four Fruit 'C'	Libby	40.0	0.1	10.0	Tr	Tr
Four Grain Muesli	Jordans	321	11.2	59.2	6.0	9.2
Four Seasons Luxury Pizza, each	Birds Eye Gino Ginelli	600	31.0	87.0	16.5	n/a
Fox's Glacier Fruits	Rowntree Mackintosh	368	nil	98.2	nil	n/a
Fox's Glacier Mints	Rowntree Mackintosh	371	nil	99.0	nil	n/a

All amounts given per 100g/100ml unless otherwise stated

Product	Brand	Calories kcal	Protein (g)	Carbo-hydrate (g)	Fat (g)	Dietary Fibre (g)
Frankfurters						
Frappe, ready to drink	Nescafe	274	9.5	3.0	25.0	0.1
Freaky Foot, each	Wall's	64.0	2.7	7.3	2.7	nil
Fred Bear Beans & Pasta Shapes	Crosse & Blackwell	90.0	1.5	12.0	4.0	n/a
Freedent Mint Chewing Gum	Wrigley	81.0	3.4	15.8	0.5	3.4
French Beans: see Green Beans/French Beans		306	nil	2.4	nil	nil
French Beef Bourguignon Microwaveable Snack	Campbell's	89.0	4.7	7.4	4.8	1.1
French Bourguignon Cook-In-Sauce	Homepride	46.0	0.7	9.5	n/a	n/a
French Bread Pizza: see flavours						
French Brie	St Ivel	297	19.0	Tr	24.5	nil
French Brie Cheese with Garlic & Herb	St Ivel	373	19.0	Tr	33.0	nil

158

French Brie Royale	St Ivel	364	19.0	Tr	32.0	nil
French Chaumes	St Ivel	303	19.5	Tr	25.0	n/a
French Dressing original	Kraft	649	0.3	0.1	72.1	nil
		496	Tr	5.0	54.0	n/a
French Fancies, each	Mr Kipling	102	0.8	19.8	2.7	n/a
French Fries, per portion						
regular	McDonald's	236	3.0	24.8	14.5	2.3
medium	McDonald's	335	4.3	35.2	20.6	3.2
large	McDonald's	472	6.0	49.6	29.0	4.6
French Fries, Gold Standard:						
crinkle cut	McCain	131	2.6	21.0	4.1	2.2
straight cut	McCain	132	2.4	21.9	3.9	2.3
French Mix Vegetables	Ross	21.0	1.7	5.1	0.1	1.8
French Mushroom & Garlic Soup	Campbell's	55.0	0.8	3.9	0.3	0.3
French Mustard	Burgess	144	6.8	12.6	6.0	0.2
	Colman's	104	6.3	n/a	7.0	n/a

All amounts given per 100g/100ml unless otherwise stated

Product	Brand	Calories kcal	Protein (g)	Carbo- hydrate (g)	Fat (g)	Dietary Fibre (g)
French Onion Soup	Baxters	24.0	0.9	5.4	Tr	Tr
	Heinz	24.0	0.5	5.2	0.1	0.3
French Roule	St Ivel	333	9.0	Tr	33.0	n/a
French Sandwich Cake	Lyons	361	3.3	58.0	14.6	0.9
French Style Yogurt: *see also flavours*						
French Style Yogurt, all varieties	Eden Vale	101	3.8	15.1	3.2	n/a
French Vinaigrette	Flora	69.0	Tr	0.2	8.0	n/a
French White Asparagus Soup	Campbell's	59.0	0.7	6.1	3.6	0.2
Fresh Fruit Salad, per pack	Boots Shapers	55.0	n/a	n/a	n/a	n/a
Fresh Garden Mint Sauce	Colman's	15.0	1.3	n/a	0.1	n/a
Fresh Juice Orange Maid Mivvi, each	Lyons Maid	61.0	0.3	14.5	Tr	n/a
Fried Bread: *see Bread, fried*						

Fromage frais (see also flavours)						
fruit		131	6.8	13.8	5.8	Tr
plain		113	6.8	5.7	7.1	nil
very low fat		58.0	7.7	6.8	0.2	Tr
	Delight	42.0	7.0	3.5	Tr	n/a
Frosties	Kellogg's	380	5.0	89.0	0.5	0.6
Fruit & Almond Slices	Lyons	326	4.1	57.1	10.6	2.4
Fruit 'n' Fibre	Kellogg's	360	9.0	69.0	5.0	7.0
Fruit & Fibre Muesli	Boots	325	12.0	51.0	9.5	14.0
Fruit & Hazelnut Ostlers	Lyons	406	5.7	54.2	20.0	5.6
Fruit & Nut Bran	Weetabix	315	12.5	49.3	7.5	18.6
Fruit & Nut Chewy Bar	Boots	403	7.3	54.0	19.0	5.3
Fruit & Nut Chocolate	Cadbury Rowntree Mackintosh	495	8.6	57.1	27.7	n/a
		477	6.8	58.3	25.7	n/a
Fruit & Nut Cookies, diabetic	Boots	414	5.9	57.0	22.0	4.7

All amounts given per 100g/100ml unless otherwise stated

Product	Brand	Calories kcal	Protein (g)	Carbohydrate (g)	Fat (g)	Dietary Fibre (g)
Fruit & Nut Harvest Chewy Bar, each	Quaker	108	1.9	15.4	4.3	0.8
Fruit & Nut Ice Cream	Wall's Dream	140	3.1	16.4	7.4	n/a
Fruit & Nut Milk Chocolate, diabetic	Boots	441	9.4	51.0	28.0	2.3
Fruit Burst Drinks (Del Monte): *see flavours*						
Fruit Cake						
plain, retail		354	5.1	57.9	12.9	N
rich, recipe		341	3.8	59.6	11.0	1.7
rich, iced		356	4.1	62.7	11.4	1.7
wholemeal		363	6.0	52.8	15.7	2.4
Fruit Club Biscuits	Jacob's	475	5.2	62.0	24.8	1.3
Fruit Cocktail						
canned in juice		57.0	0.4	14.8	Tr	1.0
canned in syrup		77.0	0.4	20.1	Tr	1.0
diabetic	Boots	26.0	0.2	6.4	Tr	1.4
Fruit Fromage Frais,						

162

creamy	Chambourcy	122	5.8	16.2	4.2	n/a
very low fat	Chambourcy	83.0	6.8	13.9	0.4	n/a
Fruit Gums		172	1.0	44.8	nil	nil
Fruit Instant Whip, made up, per serving	Bird's	137	4.1	20.0	5.1	n/a
Fruit Jaspers	McVitie's	499	5.4	65.6	23.6	3.4
Fruit Loaf	Mothers Pride	302	10.0	49.4	7.0	2.2
Fruit Loaf Mix, made up, per serving	Homepride	122	2.0	19.0	4.0	n/a
Fruit Mousse		137	4.5	18.0	5.7	N
Fruit Pastilles	Rowntree Mackintosh	329	4.1	83.3	nil	n/a
Fruit Pie, one crust		186	2.0	28.7	7.9	1.7
pastry top & bottom		260	3.0	34.0	13.3	1.8
individual		369	4.3	56.7	15.5	N
wholemeal, one crust		183	2.6	26.6	8.1	2.7
Fruit Pies (Lyons): *see flavours*						
Fruit Salad, homemade		19.0	1.1	3.0	0.4	1.5

All amounts given per 100g/100ml unless otherwise stated

Product	Brand	Calories kcal	Protein (g)	Carbo-hydrate (g)	Fat (g)	Dietary Fibre (g)
dried	Whitworths	195	2.1	48.7	Tr	8.9
Fruit Salad Chews, each	Trebor Bassett	15.0	n/a	3.3	0.2	n/a
Fruit Sauce	Lea & Perrins	151	1.5	36.2	Tr	n/a
Fruit Scone Mix, made up, per serving	Homepride	109	2.0	18.0	3.0	n/a
Fruit Scones, each	Sunblest	161	3.2	26.9	4.5	0.9
Fruit Shortcake	McVitie's	488	5.1	70.6	19.5	2.6
Fruit Shorties Biscuits	Boots	452	6.3	73.0	17.0	4.4
Fruit Shrewsbury Biscuits	Bronte	463	n/a	n/a	20.3	n/a
diabetic	Boots	424	4.4	61.0	22.0	2.3
Fruit Slice	Peek Frean	470	3.9	57.6	26.2	2.0
Fruit Snack Bars (Granose): see flavours						
Fruit Sponge Pudding Mix, made up, per serving	Homepride	342	4.5	75.5	14.5	n/a
Fruited Teacakes	Mothers Pride	266	9.7	50.1	4.4	2.2

each						
Fruitini Mixed Fruit	Sunblest	159	5.1	27.8	2.5	1.5
	Del Monte	58.0	0.4	15.0	0.1	n/a
Fruitini Peaches	Del Monte	58.0	0.4	15.0	0.1	n/a
Fruitini Pineapple	Del Monte	58.0	0.4	15.0	0.1	n/a
Fruits of the Forest, canned in syrup	Libby	82.0	0.4	20.2	Tr	0.5
Fruits of the Forest Cheesecake	McVitie's	335	4.9	30.6	21.6	0.4
Fruits of the Forest Jam, reduced calorie	Heinz Weight Watchers	125	0.4	33.0	Tr	1.8
Fruits of the Forest Pavlova	McVitie's	313	2.4	41.5	15.3	Tr
Fruits of the Forest Yogurt thick & creamy	Boots Shapers	44.0	4.6	6.7	0.1	0.6
	Boots	114	5.0	18.0	2.9	n/a
Fruity Sauce	Branston	117	0.9	25.6	0.2	1.1
	Colman's	95.0	0.9	n/a	0.2	n/a
	HP	117	1.1	27.0	0.6	n/a
Frusli Bar with apricot & almond	Jordans	388	7.3	62.5	13.8	4.0

All amounts given per 100g/100ml unless otherwise stated

Product	Brand	Calories kcal	Protein (g)	Carbo-hydrate (g)	Fat (g)	Dietary Fibre (g)
with raisin & hazelnut	Jordans	425	7.3	58.5	19.6	4.0
Fudge	Cadbury	440	3.4	72.1	17.2	n/a
Fudge Instant Whip, made up, per serving	Bird's	137	4.1	20.0	5.1	n/a
Fudge Slice	California Cake & Cookie Co.	438	5.5	69.0	22.0	n/a

Galaxy	Mars	518	9.0	56.6	30.0	n/a
Gammon: see Bacon, gammon						

Gammon Hawaii Cook In The Pot Microwave Mix, as sold	Crosse & Blackwell	372	2.7	83.0	3.2	0.4
Garden Pea with Mint Soup	Baxters	32.0	1.6	6.3	0.3	1.8
Garden Peas 1oz/28g minted premium choice	Birds Eye / Ross / Ross	15.0 / 68.0 / 68.0	1.5 / 5.1 / 5.1	Tr / 14.4 / 14.4	2.0 / 0.9 / 0.9	n/a / 4.6 / 4.6
Garden Peas & Baby Carrots in Honey Glaze	Ross	100	3.3	10.6	6.6	3.8
Garden Vegetable Soup	Crosse & Blackwell	39.0	1.0	7.2	0.7	0.9
Garibaldi Biscuits	Crawfords	408	4.0	70.6	9.4	4.2
Garlic, raw		98.0	7.9	16.3	0.6	4.1
Garlic & Chive Sauce	Heinz	305	1.1	9.2	29.3	0.3
Garlic & Herb Prawnnaise	Lyons	210	4.5	5.8	18.9	n/a
Garlic & Mint Dip, per pack	Kavli	350	6.9	6.0	33.3	n/a

All amounts given per 100g/100ml unless otherwise stated

Product	Brand	Calories kcal	Protein (g)	Carbo-hydrate (g)	Fat (g)	Dietary Fibre (g)
Garlic & Spring Onion Sauce	Lea & Perrins	74.0	1.4	16.0	0.5	n/a
Garlic Butter Flavour Rice	Batchelors	372	8.8	77.6	4.5	n/a
Garlic Dip, per pack	Kavli	350	6.9	6.0	33.3	n/a
Garlic Dippits, per pack	Kavli	294	6.2	19.3	22.0	n/a
Garlic Dressing original Italian	Flora Kraft	53.0 426	Tr Tr	1.2 7.0	5.4 43.0	n/a n/a
Garlic Mayonnaise	Hellmanns	719	1.1	1.6	78.7	n/a
Garlic Pasta Magic, frozen	Green Giant	98.0	n/a	n/a	1.0	n/a
Garlic Pate, reduced calorie	Boots Shapers	174	16.0	3.0	11.0	n/a
Garlic Prawnnaise	Lyons	451	5.7	3.3	46.9	n/a
Garlic Prawns, Golden	Young's	239	9.8	23.0	12.3	0.8
Garlic Puree	Sharwood	63.0	3.4	13.3	0.3	2.4
Garlic Sauce creamed	Lea & Perrins Burgess	91.0 427	0.8 2.6	21.5 21.3	0.2 36.2	n/a nil
Gateau		337	5.7	43.4	16.8	0.4

German Mustard	Colman's	98.0	5.3	n/a	7.5	n/a
Ghee						
butter		898	Tr	Tr	99.8	nil
palm		897	Tr	Tr	99.7	nil
vegetable		898	Tr	Tr	99.8	nil
Gherkins, pickled		14.0	0.9	2.6	0.1	1.2
raw		12.0	1.0	1.8	0.1	0.8
Giant Chocolate Chip Cookies	Boots	478	5.1	62.0	25.0	2.8
Giant Ginger Cookies	Boots	481	4.9	63.0	25.0	2.1
Giant Minestrone Soup	Heinz	53.0	1.4	8.8	1.3	1.2
Gin: *see Spirits*						
Ginger, root, raw		38.0	1.4	7.2	0.6	N
Ginger & Honey Chinese Spare Rib Sauce	Sharwood	171	2.4	37.5	1.9	1.7
Ginger & Orange Sauce	Lea & Perrins	69.0	0.3	14.6	1.0	n/a
Ginger & Pear Cereal Bar,						

All amounts given per 100g/100ml unless otherwise stated

Product	Brand	Calories kcal	Protein (g)	Carbo-hydrate (g)	Fat (g)	Dietary Fibre (g)
chocolate coated	Boots	344	1.8	64.0	1.0	2.3
Ginger & Spring Onion Marinade	Sharwood	74.0	1.4	13.2	1.8	0.9
Ginger Beer	Barr	36.0	n/a	n/a	n/a	n/a
	Corona	29.0	n/a	7.7	n/a	n/a
	Schweppes	33.9	n/a	8.8	n/a	n/a
	Idris	48.0	n/a	12.7	n/a	n/a
traditional style						
Ginger Creams, diabetic	Boots	468	7.4	64.0	22.0	3.0
Ginger Fingers	Boots	439	5.6	90.0	13.0	2.0
Ginger & Pear Bar, each	Granose	110	0.7	16.4	3.2	3.1
Gingernut Biscuits	McVitie's	456	5.6	79.1	15.2	1.4
		460	5.2	75.4	15.1	1.7
Gino Ginelli Pizzas (Birds Eye): *see flavours*						
Gipsy Creams	McVitie's	514	4.9	62.8	26.9	2.6
Glacé Cherries: *see Cherries*						
Glacé Fruit Drops, diabetic	Boots	235	Tr	98.0	0.5	Tr

Glacé Ginger	Whitworths	285	0.1	74.2	0.7	n/a
Glacé Mint Drops, diabetic	Boots	233	Tr	97.0	0.3	Tr
Glacier Fruits, Fox's	Rowntree Mackintosh	368	nil	98.2	nil	n/a
Glacier Mints, Fox's	Rowntree Mackintosh	371	nil	99.0	nil	n/a
Glazed Chicken	Findus Lean Cuisine	105	10.0	9.6	3.0	1.3
Globe Artichoke: *see Artichoke, globe*						
Glucose Energy Tablets						
original	Lucozade Sport	339	nil	90.4	n/a	n/a
lemon & lime	Lucozade Sport	339	Tr	90.4	n/a	n/a
orange	Lucozade Sport	339	Tr	90.4	n/a	n/a
Goats Milk: *see under Milk*						
Gold Margarine	St Ivel	386	6.0	3.0	39.0	n/a
for cooking	St Ivel	543	0.2	1.7	59.5	n/a
lowest fat	St Ivel	273	8.3	3.6	25.0	n/a
unsalted	St Ivel	386	6.0	3.0	39.0	n/a

All amounts given per 100g/100ml unless otherwise stated

Product	Brand	Calories kcal	Protein (g)	Carbohydrate (g)	Fat (g)	Dietary Fibre (g)
Gold Ski Yogurts (Eden Vale): see flavours						
Golden Crackles	Kellogg's	380	7.0	83.0	2.0	1.0
Golden Crisp	Cadbury	490	6.4	63.6	25.3	n/a
Golden Crown spreadable	Kraft	653	0.3	1.0	72.0	nil
light	Kraft	546	0.2	1.2	60.0	nil
Golden Crunch Biscuits	Bronte	463	n/a	n/a	20.3	n/a
Golden Cup, small	Rowntree Mackintosh	456	4.9	61.6	22.8	n/a
Golden Light Oil	Napolina	900	n/a	nil	100	nil
Golden Oatmeal Crisps	Kellogg's	370	9.0	68.0	6.0	4.0
Golden Savoury Rice	Batchelors	328	8.8	73.4	3.3	n/a
Golden Seafood (Young's): see under individual products						
Golden Sweetcorn	Del Monte	101	3.0	22.2	0.6	n/a
Golden Syrup		298	0.3	79.0	nil	nil

172

Golden Syrup Bar Cake	McVitie's	384	4.4	57.7	14.7	1.2
Golden Syrup Sponge Pudding	McVities	397	5.5	57.4	16.6	1.1
	Mr Kipling	356	3.2	62.4	12.0	n/a
Golden Toffee	Rowntree Mackintosh	454	2.9	74.3	18.2	n/a
Golden Vanilla Choc Ice, each	Wall's	124	1.5	11.6	8.4	n/a
Goose, roast, meat only		319	29.3	nil	22.4	nil
Gooseberries						
raw		54.0	0.7	12.9	0.3	2.4
stewed with sugar		73.0	0.4	18.5	0.2	2.0
green, stewed without sugar		16.0	0.9	2.5	0.3	1.9
Gouda Cheese		375	24.0	Tr	31.0	nil
Goulash	Granose	53.8	4.3	8.8	0.4	0.6
Gourmet Sauces (Rakusen): see flavours						
Grainstore Wholemeal Bread	Allinson	215	10.3	35.3	3.6	8.4
Granary Bread: see Bread						

All amounts given per 100g/100ml unless otherwise stated

Product	Brand	Calories kcal	Protein (g)	Carbo-hydrate (g)	Fat (g)	Dietary Fibre (g)
Grannies Cake	Lyons	416	4.2	54.5	21.6	2.2
Granulated Sugar	Tate & Lyle	394	nil	99.9	nil	nil
Grape juice, unsweetened						
red, sparkling	Schloer	46.0	0.3	11.7	0.1	nil
white	Schloer	49.0	Tr	13.1	n/a	n/a
white, sparkling	Schloer	48.0	Tr	12.9	n/a	n/a
	Schloer	49.0	Tr	13.1	n/a	n/a
Grape Nuts	Bird's	346	10.5	79.9	0.5	n/a
Grapefruit, raw, flesh only		30.0	0.8	6.8	0.1	1.3
canned in juice		30.0	0.6	7.3	Tr	0.4
canned in syrup		60.0	0.5	15.5	Tr	0.6
Grapefruit & Orange, canned in syrup	Libby	77.0	0.5	18.8	Tr	0.3
Grapefruit & Pineapple Drink	Tango	44.0	n/a	11.8	n/a	n/a
Grapefruit 'C'	Libby	36.0	0.2	8.8	Tr	0.3
Grapefruit Drink	Britvic 55	50.0	n/a	11.9	n/a	n/a
Grapefruit Juice, unsweetened		33.0	0.4	8.3	0.1	Tr

174

	Britvic	55.0	n/a	14.6	n/a	
	Del Monte	35.0	0.5	8.8	Tr	n/a
	St Ivel Mr Juicy	41.0	0.6	10.3	0.1	n/a
	St Ivel Real	34.0	0.6	8.3	0.1	n/a
Grapes, black/white, seedless		60.0	0.4	15.4	0.1	0.7
Gravy Browning	Burgess	72.0	3.3	14.7	nil	nil
	Crosse & Blackwell	192	Tr	48.0	nil	nil
Gravy Instant Granules made up with water		462	4.4	40.6	32.5	Tr
		33.0	0.3	2.9	2.4	Tr
Greek Pastries (sweet)		322	4.7	40.0	17.0	N
Greek Yogurt: see Yogurt						
Green & Red Peppers Ragu	Brooke Bond	79.0	1.9	11.9	2.9	n/a
Green Beans/French Beans						
raw		24.0	1.9	3.2	0.5	2.2
boiled		22.0	1.8	2.9	0.5	2.4
frozen, boiled		25.0	1.7	4.7	0.1	4.1
canned		22.0	1.5	4.1	0.1	2.6

All amounts given per 100g/100ml unless otherwise stated

Product	Brand	Calories kcal	Protein (g)	Carbo-hydrate (g)	Fat (g)	Dietary Fibre (g)
Green Butterfly	Fussell's	160	8.2	11.5	9.0	n/a
Green Chilli & Garlic Poppadums	Sharwood	274	19.9	43.3	1.6	9.7
Green Label Chutney (Sharwood): *see individual flavours*						
Green Label Chutney Sauce	Sharwood	222	1.0	44.8	0.3	1.4
Green Lentils: *see Lentils*						
Green Pepper Jelly	Baxters	255	Tr	67.0	Tr	0.7
Green Peppers: *see Peppers, green*						
Greengages						
raw (weighed with stones)		34.0	0.5	8.6	Tr	1.6
stewed with sugar		107	1.3	26.9	0.1	1.5
Greens, spring: *see Spring Greens*						
Grillados, lean beef	Findus	173	16.1	2.4	11.0	0.2
Grilled Chicken Golden Lights, per pack	Golden Wonder	110	1.3	15.8	5.0	n/a

Grillsteaks, grilled						
beef, each	Birds Eye	305	22.1	0.5	23.9	Tr
	Steakhouse	165	13.0	1.0	12.0	n/a
	Ross	337	15.0	nil	30.8	n/a
lamb, each	Birds Eye	190	15.0	1.0	14.0	n/a
	Steakhouse					
prizegrills, each	Birds Eye	195	19.0	1.0	13.0	n/a
	Steakhouse					
value, each	Birds Eye	160	14.0	6.0	9.0	n/a
	Steakhouse					
Ground Rice	Whitworths	361	6.5	86.8	1.0	2.4
Groundnuts: see Peanuts						
Grouse, roast		173	31.3	nil	5.3	nil
Guavas						
raw		26.0	0.8	5.0	0.5	3.7
canned in syrup		60.0	0.4	15.7	Tr	n/a
Gumbo: see Okra						

All amounts given per 100g/100ml unless otherwise stated

Product	Brand	Calories kcal	Protein (g)	Carbo-hydrate (g)	Fat (g)	Dietary Fibre (g)
Haddock						
steamed, flesh only		98.0	22.8	nil	0.8	nil
in crumbs, fried in oil		174	21.4	3.6	8.3	0.2
smoked, steamed, flesh only		101	23.3	nil	0.9	nil
Haddock & Prawn Crumble	Ross Recipe Meal 163		8.2	14.2	8.4	0.6
Haddock Bake	Ross Recipe Meal 198		11.3	10.9	12.3	0.5
Haddock Fillet Fish Fingers, each						
	Birds Eye	50.0	3.5	5.0	2.0	n/a
	Findus	63.0	3.8	5.0	3.1	Tr
Haddock Fillets	Ross Chip Shop	241	11.1	15.1	15.4	0.6
	Ross Fish Shop	73.0	16.8	nil	0.6	n/a
breaded	Ross Fish Shop	123	14.3	15.3	0.6	0.6

smoked	Ross	77.0	17.8	nil	0.6	n/a
smoked, with butter	Birds Eye	93.0	19.0	nil	1.9	n/a
Haddock Mornay	Ross Recipe Meal	95.0	5.9	10.5	3.4	0.4
Haddock Steaklets	Findus	215	12.0	13.6	12.5	0.5
in crunchy crumb	Findus	215	12.4	16.7	11.2	0.6
Haddock Steaks	Ross Chip Shop	241	11.1	15.1	15.4	0.7
in butter sauce	Ross	93.0	9.9	3.5	4.4	0.1
in natural crumb	Ross	197	11.6	14.9	10.4	0.6
oven crispy, each	Birds Eye	230	12.0	13.0	15.0	n/a
traditional crispy, each	Birds Eye	225	12.0	14.0	14.0	n/a
Haggis, boiled		310	10.7	19.2	21.7	N
Halibut, steamed, flesh only		131	23.8	nil	4.0	nil
Ham, canned		120	18.4	nil	5.1	nil
Ham, per slice	Delight	22.0	3.6	0.7	0.5	n/a
Ham & Beef Paste	Shippams	188	n/a	n/a	n/a	n/a
Ham & Butterbean Soup	Heinz	50.0	2.5	6.6	1.5	1.8

All amounts given per 100g/100ml unless otherwise stated

Product	Brand	Calories kcal	Protein (g)	Carbo-hydrate (g)	Fat (g)	Dietary Fibre (g)
Ham & Cheese Soup, condensed	Campbell's	117	2.4	6.7	8.9	0.1
Ham & Cheese Scrunchy	Findus	256	6.4	12.6	16.0	1.1
Ham & Cheese Toast Topper	Heinz	106	8.0	8.0	4.7	0.1
Ham & Mushroom French Bread Pizza	Heinz Weight Watchers	143	10.7	14.2	4.8	2.2
Ham & Mushroom Lasagne	Boots Shapers Ready Meals	102	4.8	8.7	6.0	1.7
	Mama Mia's	112	5.1	12.7	4.7	0.5
Ham & Mushroom Luxury Pizza, each	Birds Eye Gino Ginelli	580	30.0	87.0	15.0	n/a
Ham & Mushroom Pizza	McCain Pizza Pantry	194	9.2	23.3	5.7	n/a
	McVitie's	179	7.9	27.0	5.0	1.3
Ham & Mushroom Pizza slice	McCain Pizza Pantry	176	9.1	26.8	3.8	n/a
Ham & Mushroom	Batchelors					

Tagliatelle	Microchef Meal	119	5.1	10.2	6.4	n/a
Ham & Pepper Soup	Heinz	35.0	1.2	5.9	0.7	0.4
Ham & Pineapple Croisanti	McVitie's	307	8.1	30.9	17.4	1.3
Ham & Pineapple French Bread Pizza	Findus	193	8.0	24.6	6.9	1.3
reduced calorie	Heinz Weight Watchers	147	10.7	15.2	4.8	2.1
Ham & Pineapple Micro Pizza	McCain Pizza Perfection	205	11.9	29.0	5.4	n/a
Ham & Pork, chopped, canned		275	14.4	1.4	23.6	0.3
Ham Cubes	Knorr	258	7.8	20.5	16.3	0.1
Ham, Mushroom, Peppers & Onions French Bread Pizza	Findus	203	8.0	26.0	7.5	1.5
Ham Spread	Shippams	162	n/a	n/a	n/a	n/a
Hamburger, each	McDonald's	223	12.0	31.3	6.4	2.2
Hamburger Buns		264	9.1	48.8	5.0	1.5

All amounts given per 100g/100ml unless otherwise stated

Product	Brand	Calories kcal	Protein (g)	Carbohydrate (g)	Fat (g)	Dietary Fibre (g)
Handy Wheatgerm Bread	Hovis	237	10.1	40.6	3.1	4.7
Happy Bears						
cocoa	McVitie's	465	7.5	70.5	16.8	1.8
honey	McVitie's	476	7.3	72.2	17.3	1.8
Hard Cheese, average						
reduced fat	Heinz Weight Watchers	405	24.7	0.1	34.0	nil
		297	27.0	Tr	21.0	nil
Harlequins, each	Mr Kipling	146	1.7	25.1	5.0	n/a
Haricot Beans, dried, boiled		95.0	6.6	17.2	0.5	6.1
Harvest Chewy Bars (Quaker): *see flavours*						
Harvest Crunch	Quaker	453	6.6	72.8	16.5	5.2
tropical	Quaker	479	6.9	69.3	20.8	5.8
Harvest Grain Bread	Mothers Pride	238	7.6	43.3	3.1	3.9
Harvest Thick Vegetable Soup	Crosse & Blackwell	43.0	1.6	7.9	0.6	1.1
Harvester Bread	Vitbe	230	8.2	45.7	1.6	2.6

Hash Browns	McCain Ross	190 139	3.0 2.6	24.0 23.1	9.8 4.6	n/a 1.2
Haunted House Spaghetti Shapes in Tomato Sauce	Heinz	72.0	2.2	16.2	0.3	0.7
Hawaii Gourmet Sauce	Rakusen	77.0	n/a	n/a	2.7	n/a
Hawaiian Crunch	Mornflake	390	12.0	60.0	13.0	14.0
Hazelnut Carob Coated Fruit Snack Bar, each	Granose	207	3.5	24.6	10.5	2.3
Hazelnut Fruit Snack Bar, each	Granose	100	0.1	16.7	3.0	2.2
Hazelnut Instant Chocolate Drink	Boots Shapers	342	20.0	55.0	6.2	4.5
Hazelnut Milk Chocolate, diabetic	Boots	492	7.6	51.7	36.0	1.0
Hazelnut Munchies	Rowntree Mackintosh	489	6.3	55.4	28.4	n/a
Hazelnut Pate	Granose	140	10.0	18.0	3.0	n/a

All amounts given per 100g/100ml unless otherwise stated

Product	Brand	Calories kcal	Protein (g)	Carbohydrate (g)	Fat (g)	Dietary Fibre (g)
Hazelnut Wafer	Cadbury	531	8.8	57.2	31.2	n/a
Hazelnut Yogurt	Classic Ski	99.0	5.3	15.7	2.1	n/a
Hazelnuts, kernel only		650	14.1	6.0	63.5	6.5
Healthy Balance Ketchup	Crosse & Blackwell	93.0	1.8	20.2	0.3	0.4
Heart *ox, stewed* *sheep, roast*		179 237	31.4 26.1	nil nil	5.9 14.7	nil nil
Herb & Garlic Dressing	Heinz All Seasons	305	0.5	11.4	28.6	nil
Herb Mustard, traditional	Colman's	178	7.3	n/a	8.1	n/a
Herb Pate per tub	Tartex Vessen	238 109	7.0 3.1	12.0 5.4	18.0 7.8	0.3 0.1
Herb Vinaigrette	Flora	51.0	Tr	0.5	5.4	n/a
Herbs Vegetarian Spread	Granose	266	11.2	11.2	19.6	n/a
Hermesetas Light Yogurt, all flavours	Dairy Crest	49.3	4.1	7.7	0.4	n/a

Herring						
raw		234	16.8	nil	18.5	nil
fried, flesh only		234	23.1	1.5	15.1	N
grilled, flesh only		199	20.4	nil	13.0	nil
Hibran Bread	Vitbe	219	12.6	35.0	3.2	6.8
Hickory Nuts: see Pecan Nuts						
High Bake Water Biscuits	Jacob's	387	9.8	74.6	7.5	3.5
Hi-Fibre Biscuits	Itona	440	10.0	71.0	19.0	20.0
Hi-Fibre White Bread	Windmill	225	7.4	46.4	2.0	8.6
Hi-Fibre Wholemeal Bread	Hovis	214	9.9	36.0	2.8	8.7
Hi-Juice 66	Schweppes	51.3	n/a	13.6	n/a	n/a
High Juice Orange	Boots Shapers	16.0	0.1	3.9	0.1	nil
Highland Lentil Soup	Knorr	317	17.2	51.6	6.0	7.7
Highlander's Broth	Baxters	45.0	1.6	6.7	1.5	0.7
HiLite Bran Bread	Vitbe	222	10.2	39.1	2.8	5.5
Hilo Crackers	Rakusen	342	12.1	66.0	2.0	12.0
HiOat Bran Bread	Vitbe	225	9.4	41.4	2.4	4.4

All amounts given per 100g/100ml unless otherwise stated

Product	Brand	Calories kcal	Protein (g)	Carbohydrate (g)	Fat (g)	Dietary Fibre (g)
Hob Nob Bars	McVitie's	523	6.4	61.6	27.9	2.8
Hoi Sin Chinese Spare Rib Sauce	Sharwood	182	2.8	38.3	2.4	1.9
Honey, comb in jars		281 288	0.6 0.4	74.4 76.4	4.6 nil	nil nil
Honey & Almond Crunch Bar, original	Jordans	411	9.0	48.9	20.1	5.9
Honey & Lemon Stir Fry Cook In The Pot Dry Mix, as sold	Crosse & Blackwell	457	5.8	61.4	20.9	Tr
Honey & Mixed Nuts Yogurt, low fat	Boots	100	4.7	17.0	1.9	n/a
Honey & Pecan Thick & Creamy Yogurt,	Boots	124	4.7	19.0	3.8	0.5
Honey Crunchy Cereal	Holland & Barrett	390	12.0	60.0	12.0	14.0
Honey Glazed Chicken,	Birds Eye					

per pack						
	Healthy Options	420	28.0	71.0	4.5	n/a
Honey Nut Loops	Kellogg's	380	8.0	78.0	4.0	5.0
Honey Pots Le Yogurt Actif, stirred	Chambourcy	120	5.8	15.0	4.0	0.7
Honeycomb: see Honey						
Honeydew Melon: see Melon						
Hong Kong Sweet & Sour Pork with Yangtze Special Rice	Heinz	161	6.6	17.7	7.1	0.5
Horlicks Chocolate Malted Food Drink low fat, instant	SmithKline Beecham	358	8.7	79.3	3.1	n/a
instant	Smithkline Beecham	390	11.0	75.0	7.1	n/a
Horlicks Hot Chocolate Drink, low fat, instant	SmithKline Beecham	401	18.3	66.0	8.4	n/a
Horlicks LowFat Instant Powder made up with water		373 / 51.0	17.4 / 2.4	72.9 / 10.1	3.3 / 0.5	N / Tr
Horlicks Maltlets	SmithKline					

All amounts given per 100g/100ml unless otherwise stated

Product	Brand	Calories kcal	Protein (g)	Carbo-hydrate (g)	Fat (g)	Dietary Fibre (g)
Horlicks Powder	Beecham	384	12.4	78.0	4.0	n/a
made up with whole milk		378	12.4	78.0	4.0	N
made up with semi-skimmed milk		99.0	4.2	12.7	3.9	Tr
		81.0	4.3	12.9	1.9	Tr
Horseradish, creamed	Burgess	199	2.7	21.3	10.5	2.5
Horseradish Mustard	Colman's	158	5.9	n/a	6.5	n/a
Horseradish Relish	Colman's	93.0	1.7	n/a	5.5	n/a
Horseradish sauce	Burgess	153	2.5	17.9	8.4	2.5
hot		118	2.1	11.7	6.0	2.3
Hot & Spicy French Bread Pizza	Findus	229	8.0	29.0	9.0	1.9
Hot Chilli Sauce	Heinz	106	2.6	24.0	Tr	0.1
Hot Cross Buns		310	7.4	58.5	6.8	1.7
Hot Crunch Puddings, made up, per serving, all flavours	Bird's	222	2.7	39.6	7.0	n/a
Hot Curry Paste	Sharwood	352	5.1	9.7	32.6	7.6

188

Hot Pepper Sauce	Lea & Perrins	112	1.0	24.4	1.2	n/a
Hot Pot		114	9.4	10.1	4.5	1.2
Hot Madras Curry Sauce Mix, as sold	Sharwood	239	11.9	22.9	10.8	16.6
Hot Vegetable Curry	Sharwood	77.0	1.8	9.4	3.6	2.3
Houmous: *see Hummus*						
Hovis Bread: *see flavours*						
Hovis Crackers	Nabisco	468	9.3	64.1	21.0	4.0
Hovis Digestive	Nabisco	486	6.9	67.0	22.9	2.5
HP Sauce	HP	100	1.2	24.1	0.5	n/a
HP Sauces: *see flavours*						
Hubba Bubba Bubble Gum, all flavours	Wrigley	280	nil	2.5	nil	nil
Hula Hoops: *see Potato Hoops*						
Hummus (chick pea spread)		187	7.6	11.6	12.6	2.4
Hycal Juice, ready to drink, all flavours	SmithKline Beecham	243	nil	64.7	n/a	n/a

All amounts given per 100g/100ml unless otherwise stated

Product	Brand	Calories kcal	Protein (g)	Carbo-hydrate (g)	Fat (g)	Dietary Fibre (g)
I Can't Believe It's Not Butter	Van Den Berghs	636	0.8	0.6	70.0	n/a
Ice Cream: see also flavours						
dairy vanilla		194	3.6	24.4	9.8	Tr
dairy flavoured		179	3.5	24.7	8.0	Tr
non-dairy vanilla		178	3.2	23.1	8.7	Tr
non-dairy flavoured		166	3.1	23.2	7.4	Tr
mixes		182	4.1	25.1	7.9	Tr
Ice Cream Wafers		342	10.1	78.8	0.7	N
Ice Magic, made up per serving, all flavours	Bird's	66.0	0.5	3.6	5.6	n/a
Iced Gem Biscuits	Peek Frean	481	5.2	86.3	3.3	2.0
Iced Shorties	Crawfords	470	4.8	73.4	17.2	1.6

Iced Tarts	Lyons	418	3.4	70.0	15.7	1.1
Icing Sugar	Tate & Lyle	392	nil	99.6	nil	nil
Ideal Sauce	Heinz Ploughman's	109	0.6	26.6	Tr	0.7
Indian Bombay Mix	Sharwood	442	18.1	33.2	27.2	15.5
Indian Chevda	Sharwood	500	16.2	34.2	34.1	11.0
Indian Chicken & Coconut Soup	Heinz	45.0	2.0	5.3	1.7	0.5
Indian Chicken Korma Microwaveable Snack	Campbell's	154	6.3	19.1	5.9	1.1
Indian Chicken Korma Soup	Campbell's	84.0	2.2	7.2	4.4	0.2
Indian Chicken Stir Fry Meal	Ross	83.0	5.3	13.9	1.5	1.8
Indian Chicken Tikka Masala Microwave Meal	Sharwood	148	8.0	15.3	5.9	2.4
Indian Curry Rolls	Ross	176	3.5	25.4	7.3	1.4
Indian Curry Sauce & Vegetables Stir Fry	Uncle Ben's	48.0	0.7	11.1	0.1	n/a

All amounts given per 100g/100ml unless otherwise stated

Product	Brand	Calories kcal	Protein (g)	Carbo-hydrate (g)	Fat (g)	Dietary Fibre (g)
Indian Fried Savoury Rice	Batchelors	368	8.9	67.1	9.0	n/a
Indian Medium Curry Cook-In-Sauce	Homepride	59.0	1.0	10.5	n/a	n/a
Indian Prawn Biryani Stir Fry	Ross	90.0	3.7	18.3	0.3	1.8
Indian Special Rice	Ross	118	2.8	26.1	0.8	1.3
Indian Tandoori Prawns Stir Fry	Ross	74.0	3.3	14.6	0.8	1.2
Indian Tonic Water	Schweppes	35.2	n/a	9.4	n/a	n/a
Indian Vegetable Curry Microwaveable Snack	Campbell's	72.0	2.9	13.0	1.3	1.9
Indonesian Sauce For Rice	Sharwood	38.0	3.3	5.3	0.4	0.8
Inspirations	Cadbury	500	5.9	58.6	28.5	n/a
Instant Coffee: *see Coffee*						
Instant Dessert Powder		391	2.4	60.1	17.3	1.0
made up with whole milk		111	3.1	14.8	6.3	0.2
made up with skimmed milk		84.0	3.1	14.9	3.2	0.2

Instant Milk: see brands

Instant Potato Powder

made up with water		57.0	1.5	13.5	0.1	1.0
made up with whole milk		76.0	2.4	14.8	1.2	1.0
made up with semi-skimmed milk		70.0	2.4	14.8	1.2	1.0
made up with skimmed milk		66.0	2.4	14.8	0.1	1.0
Instant Soup Powder, dried		341	6.5	64.4	14.0	N
made up with water		55.0	1.1	10.5	2.3	N

Instant Whip Desserts (Bird's): see flavours

Irish Stew						
canned	Tyne Brand	123	5.3	9.1	7.6	0.9
	Tyne Brand	81.0	4.7	7.1	4.0	n/a
Irn Bru	Barr	43.0	n/a	n/a	n/a	n/a
diet	Barr	4.1	n/a	n/a	n/a	n/a
Italian Bean & Pasta Soup	Baxters	33.0	1.7	6.6	Tr	1.7
Italian Bean Salad	Batchelors	116	5.9	22.2	1.0	n/a
Italian Beans	Heinz	95.0	5.2	15.5	1.3	6.3
Italian Bolognese Cook-In-Sauce	Homepride	63.0	1.4	12.9	n/a	n/a

All amounts given per 100g/100ml unless otherwise stated

193

Product	Brand	Calories kcal	Protein (g)	Carbohydrate (g)	Fat (g)	Dietary Fibre (g)
Italian Garlic Dressing, original	Kraft	426	Tr	7.0	43.0	n/a
Italian Lasagne Verdi Microwaveable Snack	Campbell's	144	6.9	12.9	7.5	0.7
Italian Rice Choice, as sold	Crosse & Blackwell	364	8.4	74.3	3.7	2.7
Italian Style Cottage Cheese	St Ivel Shape	70.0	13.0	3.3	0.7	n/a
Italian Style Supernoodles	Batchelors	474	7.4	56.2	26.0	n/a
Italian Tomato & Basil Soup	Heinz	36.0	0.8	7.4	0.3	1.2
Italian Tomato & Red Pepper Soup	Campbell's	51.0	1.3	8.5	1.5	0.3
Izmir Gourmet Sauce	Rakusen	53.0	n/a	n/a	2.9	n/a

Jacket Potato Cheese & Onion, half	Birds Eye	180	6.0	23.0	8.0	n/a
Jacket Scallops	Ross	117	2.8	20.7	3.2	1.5
Jacket Wedges	Ross	128	2.7	21.1	4.3	1.6
Jackfruit, raw canned, drained		88.0 104	1.3 0.5	21.4 26.3	0.3 0.3	N N
Jaffa Cakes	McVitie's	376	3.9	72.3	8.2	0.9
Jaffa Fingers, each	Mr Kipling	136	0.9	18.2	7.1	n/a
Jaffa Orange Yogurt, low fat	Boots	92.0	4.6	17.0	1.1	n/a
Jaggery		367	0.5	97.2	nil	nil
Jalapeno Bean Dip	Old El Paso	108	n/a	n/a	n/a	n/a

All amounts given per 100g/100ml unless otherwise stated

Product	Brand	Calories kcal	Protein (g)	Carbohydrate (g)	Fat (g)	Dietary Fibre (g)
Jam						
fruit with edible seeds		261	0.6	69.0	nil	N
stone fruit		261	0.4	69.3	nil	N
reduced sugar		123	0.5	31.9	0.1	N
Jam Doughnuts: see Doughnuts						
Jam Mini Rolls, each	Cadbury	114	1.5	17.6	4.7	n/a
Jam Rings	Crawfords	473	4.9	70.6	18.6	1.7
Jam Roly Poly	McVitie's	395	5.5	51.6	18.9	1.0
Jam Sponge Puddings	Lyons	316	3.0	67.6	5.6	0.7
Jam Swiss Roll, boxed	Mr Kipling	211	2.5	48.1	2.3	n/a
Jam Tarts, recipe		380	3.3	62.0	14.9	1.6
retail	Lyons	368	3.3	63.4	13.0	N
	Mr Kipling	399	3.8	64.9	15.6	2.3
each		127	1.5	20.2	5.0	n/a
Jamaica Ginger Bar Cake	McVitie's	380	4.1	55.8	14.8	0.9
Jamboree Mallows	Peek Frean	392	3.6	67.0	9.9	1.3
Japanese Beef Oriental						

Stir Fry	Ross	65.0	6.0	10.4	0.7	1.7
Jelly, made with water		61.0	1.2	15.1	nil	nil
Jelly Crystals: *see flavours*						
Jellytots	Rowntree Mackintosh	342	nil	91.1	nil	n/a
Juicy Fruit Chewing Gum	Wrigley	306	nil	2.4	nil	nil
Julienne Salad	Eden Vale	140	3.2	9.3	10.3	n/a

Kale: *see Curly Kale*

Kashmir Mild Curry Sauce	Colman's	80.0	0.8	n/a	4.9	n/a
Kashmir Mild Curry						

All amounts given per 100g/100ml unless otherwise stated

Product	Brand	Calories kcal	Protein (g)	Carbo-hydrate (g)	Fat (g)	Dietary Fibre (g)
Sauce Mix	Sharwood	180	10.7	12.5	9.7	28.8
Kashmiri Beef Curry, per pack	Birds Eye Healthy Options	410	24.0	69.0	6.0	n/a
Kashmiri Chicken Curry	Findus Lean Cuisine	110	7.0	14.7	2.6	1.6
Kedgeree		166	14.2	10.5	7.9	Tr
Keg Bitter: see Beer						
Ketchup, tomato		98.0	2.1	24.0	Tr	0.9
Kidney						
lamb, fried		155	24.6	nil	6.3	nil
ox, stewed		172	25.6	nil	7.7	nil
pig, stewed		153	24.4	nil	6.1	nil
Kidney Beans: see Red Kidney Beans						
King Cones (Lyons Maid): see flavours						
King Prawns						
breaded	Lyons	266	16.8	15.7	15.6	n/a
Golden	Young's	241	8.7	15.6	16.3	0.7

Kings Acre Cider	HP Bulmer	53.0	n/a	n/a	n/a	n/a
Kingsize Cheesecake Mix, made up	Lyons Tetley	270	5.5	30.1	13.8	n/a
Kingsmill Bread	Allied Bakeries	233	8.6	45.1	2.0	2.3
Kingsmill Rolls, each	Allied Bakeries	123	3.7	20.6	2.6	0.8
Kipper Fillets with Butter	Birds Eye	220	17.5	nil	16.6	n/a
	Young's	184	17.3	nil	12.8	n/a
Kippers, baked, flesh only		205	25.5	nil	11.4	nil
Kiri Sparkling Apple Juice	H P Bulmer	38.0	n/a	n/a	n/a	n/a
diet Kiri	H P Bulmer	3.75	n/a	n/a	n/a	n/a
Kit Kat	Rowntree Mackintosh	501	7.2	63.0	26.2	n/a
Kiwi Fruit		49.0	1.1	10.6	0.5	1.9
canned in syrup	Libby	69.0	n/a	n/a	Tr	n/a
Kohl Rabi, raw		23.0	1.6	3.7	0.2	2.2
boiled		18.0	1.2	3.1	0.2	1.9
Kola Drops, each	Trebor Bassett	17.0	n/a	4.5	n/a	n/a

All amounts given per 100g/100ml unless otherwise stated

Product	Brand	Calories kcal	Protein (g)	Carbohydrate (g)	Fat (g)	Dietary Fibre (g)
Kola Kubes, each	Trebor Bassett	17.0	n/a	4.5	n/a	n/a
Korma Classic Curry Sauce canned	Homepride	82.0	1.4	10.2	n/a	n/a
jar	Homepride	113	2.4	13.0	n/a	n/a
Korma Curry Sauce	Sharwood	88.0	2.2	8.5	5.0	2.3
Korma Mild Curry Sauce	Colman's	73.0	2.5	n/a	4.5	n/a
Krackawheat	McVitie's	518	8.3	61.0	25.8	4.9
Krona Dairy Spread, Gold/Silver	Van Den Berghs	638	0.3	1.9	70.0	n/a
spreadable	Van Den Berghs	548	0.3	1.8	60.0	n/a
Kung Po Prawns with Special Egg Rice	Heinz	127	5.9	17.0	3.9	0.7

L

Lady's Fingers: see Okra

Lager, bottled		29.0	0.2	1.5	Tr	nil
Lager & Lime	Barr	24.0	n/a	n/a	n/a	n/a
Lamb, breast						
lean & fat, roast		410	19.1	nil	37.1	nil
lean only, roast		252	25.6	nil	16.6	nil
Lamb, chops						
loin, lean & fat, grilled		355	23.5	nil	29.0	nil
loin, lean only, grilled		222	27.8	nil	12.3	nil
Lamb, cutlets						
lean & fat, grilled		370	23.0	nil	30.9	nil
lean only, grilled		222	27.8	nil	12.3	nil

All amounts given per 100g/100ml unless otherwise stated

Product	Brand	Calories kcal	Protein (g)	Carbo-hydrate (g)	Fat (g)	Dietary Fibre (g)
Lamb, leg						
lean & fat, roast		266	26.1	nil	17.9	nil
lean only, roast		191	29.4	nil	8.1	nil
Lamb, scrag & neck						
lean & fat, stewed		292	25.6	nil	21.1	nil
lean only, stewed		253	27.8	nil	15.7	nil
Lamb, shoulder						
lean & fat, roast		316	19.9	nil	26.3	nil
lean only, roast		196	23.8	nil	11.2	nil
Lamb & Dumpling Stewpot	Mr Brain's	106	5.6	8.6	5.8	n/a
Lamb & Vegetable Casserole	Heinz Lunchbowl	86.0	5.1	8.5	3.5	1.8
Lamb Cubes	Knorr	319	11.4	25.3	19.8	0.4
Lamb Curry, canned	Tyne Brand	105	6.0	7.2	6.0	n/a
Lamb Grillsteak, each	Birds Eye	190	15.0	1.0	14.0	n/a
Lamb Hotpot Mix, as sold	Colman's	286	9.1	n/a	1.5	n/a
Lamb Hotpot Pot Meal	Boots Shapers	65.0	5.1	7.0	2.0	n/a

Lamb Korma	Boots Shapers	87.0	5.8	9.2	3.3	0.8
Lamb Pasanda with Lemon Basmati Rice, per pack	Birds Eye MenuMaster	665	31.0	62.0	34.0	n/a
Lamb Ragout Cook In The Pot Dry Mix, as sold	Crosse & Blackwell	346	10.6	59.5	7.3	2.2
Lamb Rogan Josh	Findus Dinner Supreme	193	8.6	17.2	10.5	1.7
Lamb Tikka Masala	Findus Lean Cuisine	112	8.0	14.4	2.5	1.7
Lancashire Cheese		373	23.3	0.1	31.0	nil
Lancashire Hotpot						
canned	Tyne Brand	82.0	5.5	7.2	3.5	n/a
per pack	Birds Eye MenuMaster	265	13.0	30.0	11.0	n/a
Lard		891	Tr	Tr	99.0	nil
Lasagne, frozen, cooked	Batchelors Microchef Meal	102	5.0	12.8	3.8	N
per pack	Birds Eye Menu	143	6.9	12.4	7.6	n/a

All amounts given per 100g/100ml unless otherwise stated

Product	Brand	Calories kcal	Protein (g)	Carbo-hydrate (g)	Fat (g)	Dietary Fibre (g)
	Master Findus Dinner Supreme Mama Mia's	375	20.0	33.0	19.0	n/a
		120	7.0	10.9	5.4	0.9
		117	6.5	13.3	4.5	0.6
Lasagne (pasta)						
egg, raw standard, raw cooked	Buitoni Buitoni Dolmio	342	13.4	68.0	1.8	3.5
		348	13.0	70.0	1.8	3.4
		231	8.8	44.6	1.9	n/a
Lasagne al Forno, per pack	Birds Eye	515	25.0	48.0	26.0	n/a
Lasagne Bolognese	Dolmio Ready Meals	139	5.8	11.3	8.2	n/a
Lasagne Vegetale	Dolmio Ready Meals	100	2.6	11.3	5.2	n/a
Lasagne Verdi	Findus Lean Cuisine	84.0	7.1	9.2	2.1	1.2
Lattice Oven Fries	McCain	210	2.0	31.8	9.2	n/a
Lattice Treacle Tart	Mr Kipling	351	4.0	64.7	10.3	n/a
Le Grand Desserts						

chocolate/vanilla	Chamboury	134	3.6	19.7	4.5	0.3
strawberry/vanilla	Chamboury	131	3.8	19.8	4.1	0.2
Le Yogurt (Chamboury): *see also flavours*						
Le Yogurt Actif set, all fruit flavours	Chamboury	104	4.6	13.3	3.6	nil
Le Yogurt French Style						
fruit flavour varieties	Chamboury	85.0	4.4	14.8	0.9	nil
fruit & flower varieties	Chamboury	85.0	4.4	14.8	0.9	nil
rich & creamy varieties	Chamboury	113	4.1	13.7	4.6	nil
natural	Chamboury	57.0	5.2	7.1	0.9	Tr
Leaf Spinach, premium choice	Ross	19.0	2.8	3.5	0.5	2.8
Lean Beef Casserole, per pack	Birds Eye Healthy Options	350	21.0	54.0	7.5	n/a
Lean Beef Lasagne per pack	Birds Eye Healthy Options	345	29.0	38.0	9.5	n/a
	Findus Lean Cuisine	91.0	6.2	11.5	2.2	1.1

All amounts given per 100g/100ml unless otherwise stated

Product	Brand	Calories kcal	Protein (g)	Carbo-hydrate (g)	Fat (g)	Dietary Fibre (g)
Lean Beef Madras with Turmeric Rice	Findus Lean Cuisine	99.0	6.7	14.0	1.8	1.5
Lean Cuisine (Findus): see flavours						
Leeks, boiled		21.0	1.2	2.6	0.7	1.7
Leicester Cheese		401	24.3	0.1	33.7	nil
Lemon & Cream Frousse	Gold Ski	163	4.8	18.8	8.1	n/a
Lemon & Garlic Sauce	Lea & Perrins	91.0	0.8	21.5	0.2	n/a
Lemon & Ginger Sauce & Vegetables Stir Fry	Uncle Ben's	61.0	0.5	13.0	0.7	n/a
Lemon & Lime Club Biscuits	Jacob's	505	5.6	63.0	27.4	0.8
Lemon & Lime Drink sparkling	Quosh	29.0	n/a	7.6	n/a	n/a
	Jusoda	28.0	n/a	n/a	n/a	n/a
sparkling, low calorie	Diet Jusoda	1.2	n/a	n/a	n/a	n/a
Lemon & Sultana Devonshire Cheese Cake	St Ivel	276	6.7	29.8	15.2	n/a
Lemon Bakewells, each	Mr Kipling	204	2.1	30.9	8.8	n/a

Lemon Barley Water	Robinsons	22.0	Tr	n/a	Tr	n/a
Lemon Bon Bons, each	Trebor Bassett	27.0	n/a	5.9	0.4	n/a
Lemon Brulee, each	Birds Eye	199	1.1	36.0	6.7	n/a
Lemon Carob Coated Fruit Bar, each	Granose	162	2.7	30.2	3.3	2.3
Lemon Cheesecake Mix, made up, per serving	Homepride	240	3.0	27.0	13.0	n/a
Lemon Chicken with Yangtze Special Rice	Heinz	146	8.1	19.7	3.9	0.6
Lemon Creme Sundae Yogurt	St Ivel Shape	42.0	4.9	5.5	0.1	n/a
Lemon Curd, starch base		283	0.6	62.7	5.1	0.2
Lemon Curd Tart	Lyons	416	3.5	66.2	17.1	1.2
Lemon Drink, diluted sparkling	Quosh St Clements	20.0 43.0	n/a n/a	5.2 n/a	n/a n/a	n/a n/a
Lemon Flavour Jelly Crystals	Dietade	7.0	1.6	0.2	n/a	n/a
Lemon Flavour Sandwich Wafers, Diabetic	Boots	497	11.0	57.0	25.0	2.5

All amounts given per 100g/100ml unless otherwise stated

Product	Brand	Calories kcal	Protein (g)	Carbo-hydrate (g)	Fat (g)	Dietary Fibre (g)
Lemon Hubba Bubba Bubble Gum	Wrigley	280	nil	2.5	nil	n/a
Lemon Iced Gingerbread	California Cake & Cookie Co.	291	5.7	48.5	9.6	1.1
Lemon Juice, fresh		7.0	0.3	1.6	Tr	0.1
Lemon Juice Drink undiluted	Hycal / PLJ	243 / 25.0	nil / 0.3	64.7 / 2.3	n/a / n/a	n/a / n/a
Lemon Mayonnaise	Hellmanns	720	1.0	1.5	78.9	n/a
Lemon Meringue Crunch Mix, made up, per serving	Homepride	234	2.5	36.0	10.0	n/a
Lemon Meringue Gateau	McVities	336	2.3	34.2	21.1	Tr
Lemon Meringue Pie, recipe		319	4.5	45.9	14.4	0.7
Lemon Meringues	Lyons	385	3.9	66.6	13.3	1.0
Lemon, Orange, Hazelnut & Raisin Yogurt, low fat	Holland & Barrett	105	5.4	17.3	0.8	0.2
Lemon Pie Filling Mix	Royal	147	1.0	28.0	5.0	n/a
Lemon Puffs	Huntley &					

Lemon Rice	Palmer	518	5.0	60.0	30.3	1.5
Lemon Slices, each	Sharwood	358	7.5	71.9	3.2	1.3
	Mr Kipling	114	1.1	16.4	5.3	n/a
Lemon Sole fried in crumbs		216	16.1	9.3	13.0	0.4
steamed		91.0	20.6	nil	0.9	nil
Lemon Sole Goujons, Golden	Young's	246	10.9	26.4	11.2	1.1
Lemon Sorbet		131	0.9	34.2	Tr	nil
Lemon Souffle Dessert, each	Birds Eye	132	2.1	23.3	3.9	n/a
Lemon Squash, undiluted low calorie	St Clements	142	Tr	33.3	0.2	n/a
	Dietade	7.0	n/a	0.4	n/a	n/a
Lemon Torte	Boots Shapers	195	4.4	21.0	11.0	1.0
Lemonade, bottled	Barr	21.0	Tr	5.6	nil	nil
	Corona	27.0	n/a	n/a	n/a	n/a
	R Whites	23.0	n/a	6.2	n/a	n/a
	Barr	20.0	n/a	5.3	n/a	n/a
low calorie	Corona	0.9	n/a	n/a	n/a	n/a
	Corona	0.5	nil	nil	n/a	n/a

All amounts given per 100g/100ml unless otherwise stated

Product	Brand	Calories kcal	Protein (g)	Carbohydrate (g)	Fat (g)	Dietary Fibre (g)
traditional style	R Whites	0.5	n/a	nil	n/a	n/a
	Idris	27.0	n/a	7.0	n/a	n/a
Lemonade Shandy	Top Deck	25.0	n/a	4.8	n/a	n/a
Lemons, whole, without pips		19.0	1.0	3.2	0.3	N
Lentil & Bacon Soup	Baxters	56.0	2.0	7.6	1.0	0.9
Lentil & Carrot Soup	Heinz	26.0	1.3	4.9	0.1	0.8
Lentil & Vegetable Casserole	Granose	100	3.0	12.0	4.0	1.7
Lentil Dhal	Holland & Barrett	105	6.0	15.5	2.4	1.8
Lentil Roast	Granose	336	30.4	45.8	4.7	n/a
Lentil Soup	Heinz Whole Soup	99.0	4.4	12.7	3.8	1.1
condensed	Campbell's	40.0	2.4	7.4	0.1	1.5
	Granny's Soups	59.0	3.1	10.0	0.8	1.5
Lentils *green/brown, boiled*		105	8.8	16.9	0.7	3.8

red, boiled		100	7.6	17.5	0.4	1.9
Lettuce, average, raw		14.0	0.8	1.7	0.5	0.9
Lhabia & Mushroom Bhajee	Sharwood	94.0	3.5	11.4	4.1	2.1
Light Brown Soft Sugar	Tate & Lyle	384	Tr	95.8	nil	nil
Lightly Salted Golden Lights, per pack	Golden Wonder	111	1.1	15.7	5.3	n/a
Lightly Salted Thick & Crunchy Crisps, per pack	Golden Wonder	149	1.8	14.6	9.6	n/a
Lima Beans: see Butter Beans						
Lime Cordial, diluted	Britvic	17.0	n/a	4.6	n/a	n/a
	Quosh	18.0	n/a	4.8	n/a	n/a
Lime Crusha	Burgess	115	nil	44.8	nil	nil
Lime Juice Cordial, undiluted		112	Tr	27.0	nil	nil
Lime Pickle	Sharwood	51.0	2.6	2.1	3.6	3.3
Lime Squash	St Clements	132	0.2	30.5	0.2	n/a
Limeade	Corona	23.0	n/a	6.0	n/a	n/a
Limeade & Lager	Top Deck	31.0	n/a	6.9	n/a	n/a

All amounts given per 100g/100ml unless otherwise stated

Product	Brand	Calories kcal	Protein (g)	Carbo-hydrate (g)	Fat (g)	Dietary Fibre (g)
Lincoln Biscuits	Peek Frean	486	6.3	65.8	23.8	2.5
	McVitie's	508	5.8	67.1	23.5	2.0
diabetic	Boots	468	21.0	51.0	20.0	2.4
Linguine	Napolina	320	11.5	68.4	1.5	5.6
Lion Bar	Rowntree Mackintosh	481	6.5	65.9	23.1	n/a
mini	Rowntree Mackintosh	496	6.5	69	23.5	n/a
Liquorice Allsorts	Trebor Bassett	313	3.9	74.1	2.2	N
		358	2.1	77.6	4.7	2.0
Liquorice Chewing Gum, PK	Wrigley	352	nil	Tr	nil	n/a
Liquorice Toffees	Itona	395	0.6	66.5	15.2	n/a
each	Trebor Bassett	31.0	n/a	4.5	1.4	n/a
Liquorice Torpedoes	Trebor Bassett	370	3.5	nil	0.4	1.0
Lite Fruit Mousse, made up per serving, all flavours	Bird's	46.0	2.0	6.6	1.4	n/a
Liver						
calf, fried		254	26.9	7.3	13.2	0.2

chicken, fried		194	20.7	3.4	10.9	0.2
lamb, fried		232	22.9	3.9	14.0	0.1
ox, stewed		198	24.8	3.6	9.5	Tr
pig, stewed		189	25.6	3.6	8.1	Tr
Liver & Bacon Casserole						
per pack	Birds Eye MenuMaster	410	24.0	43.0	17.0	n/a
	Mr Brain's	139	7.3	12.3	5.7	n/a
	Campbell's	74.0	4.6	8.3	2.8	0.8
canned						
Liver & Bacon Casserole						
Cooking Mix	Colman's	295	10.0	n/a	1.2	n/a
Liver & Bacon Paste	Shippams	181	n/a	n/a	n/a	n/a
Liver Pate		316	13.1	1.0	28.9	Tr
low fat		191	18.0	2.8	12.0	Tr
Liver Sausage		310	12.9	4.3	26.9	0.5
Liver with Onions &	Birds Eye					
Gravy, per pack	MenuMaster	150	18.0	6.0	6.0	n/a
Lobster, boiled		119	22.1	nil	3.4	nil
Lobster Bisque	Baxters	51.0	2.6	5.3	2.4	0.1

All amounts given per 100g/100ml unless otherwise stated

Product	Brand	Calories kcal	Protein (g)	Carbohydrate (g)	Fat (g)	Dietary Fibre (g)
Lobster in Brine	Young's	63.0	14.5	nil	0.5	n/a
Lockets	Mars	359	nil	95.8	nil	nil
Long Grain & Wild Rice	Uncle Ben's	112	3.7	23.5	0.5	n/a
Long Grain Rice	Uncle Ben's	115	2.6	25.6	0.3	n/a
	Whitworths	361	6.5	86.8	1.0	2.4
canned, 3 min	Uncle Ben's	101	2.3	23.0	0.6	n/a
frozen	Uncle Ben's	132	3.0	30.3	0.7	n/a
Low Fat Spread (see also flavours)						
	Kerrygold	390	5.8	0.5	40.5	nil
		380	n/a	n/a	n/a	n/a
Lucozade						
original	SmithKline Beecham	67.0	Tr	18.0	nil	nil
all other flavours	SmithKline Beecham	72.0	nil	19.3	nil	nil
sport, all flavours	SmithKline Beecham	72.0	Tr	19.3	nil	nil
	SmithKline Beecham	26.0	Tr	9.9	nil	nil
Lunchbar (Boots Shapers): see flavours						
Luncheon Meat, canned		313	12.6	5.5	26.9	0.3

Luxury Fruited Buns, each	Sunblest	158	4.2	27.2	3.6	1.5
Luxury Vanilla Dairy Ice Cream	Boots Shapers	83.0	3.1	11.0	3.3	Tr
Lychees raw		58.0	0.9	14.3	0.1	0.7
canned in syrup		68.0	0.4	17.7	Tr	0.5
Lymeswold Cheese, blue/white		425	15.6	Tr	40.3	nil

M & Ms, chocolate	Mars	475	5.3	7.0	21.0	1.0
peanut	Mars	494	10.6	57.7	26.1	3.6
Macadamia Nuts, salted		748	7.9	4.8	77.6	5.3
Macaroni, boiled		86.0	3.0	18.5	0.5	0.9

All amounts given per 100g/100ml unless otherwise stated

Product	Brand	Calories kcal	Protein (g)	Carbo-hydrate (g)	Fat (g)	Dietary Fibre (g)
Macaroni, creamed	Ambrosia	92.0	4.0	14.6	1.9	n/a
Macaroni Cheese per pack	Birds Eye MenuMaster	178	7.3	13.6	10.8	0.5
	Findus Dinner	540	24.0	51.0	28.0	n/a
canned	Supreme	177	7.4	16.9	9.3	0.1
	Heinz	100	3.6	10.5	4.8	0.3
Macaroni Cheese Sauce Mix, as sold	Colman's	407	20.0	n/a	18.0	n/a
Macaroni Cheese with Ham & Vegetables	Heinz Weight Watchers	89.0	5.1	11.2	2.6	0.8
Macaroni Provencale Snack Pot	Boots Shapers	80.0	5.2	8.9	2.9	2.2
McChicken Sandwich, each	McDonald's	372	18.3	44.8	14.5	2.9
Mackerel, fried, flesh only		188	21.5	nil	11.3	nil
Madeira Cake	Mr Kipling	393	5.4	58.4	16.9	0.9
Madeira Loaf Mix, made up,		325	4.6	47.1	14.5	n/a

per serving						
Madeira Wine Gravy Sauce, dry, as sold	Homepride	136	2.0	21.0	5.0	n/a
	Crosse & Blackwell Bonne Cuisine	358	8.4	63.1	8.0	1.5
Madras Classic Curry Sauce						
can	Homepride	54.0	2.2	9.6	n/a	n/a
jar	Homepride	90.0	1.8	11.8	n/a	n/a
Madras Curry Sauce, canned	Sharwood	100	1.7	6.9	7.3	1.6
Madras Medium Curry Cooking Mix	Colman's	278	6.4	n/a	5.0	n/a
Madras Medium Curry Sauce	Colman's	42.0	1.0	n/a	0.6	n/a
Madras Mild Veg Curry	Holland & Barrett	83.0	2.8	11.5	3.54	0.9
Magnifico Cornetto, each	Wall's	320	5.0	39.0	17.0	n/a
Magnum Choc Bars, each						
dark	Wall's	290	4.0	27.0	19.5	n/a
white	Wall's	290	4.0	27.0	19.5	n/a
Main Course Soups (Campbell's): *see flavours*						

All amounts given per 100g/100ml unless otherwise stated

Product	Brand	Calories kcal	Protein (g)	Carbo-hydrate (g)	Fat (g)	Dietary Fibre (g)
Major Green Chutney	Sharwood	216	0.3	57.5	0.2	0.8
Malaysian Chicken Satay Microwave Meal	Sharwood	130	8.2	14.7	4.7	1.8
Malaysian Mild Paste	Sharwood	229	3.8	8.0	20.2	6.9
Malaysian Mild Sauce	Sharwood	148	1.9	8.0	12.0	3.6
Malaysian Mild Vegetable Curry	Sharwood	148	1.9	8.0	12.0	3.6
Malaysian Salad	Eden Vale	214	3.3	10.0	18.1	n/a
Malaysian Satay Marinade	Sharwood	131	2.7	20.7	3.9	2.9
Malaysian Satay Sauce	Sharwood	632	17.9	14.5	55.8	6.0
Malaysian Sauce for Rice	Sharwood	99.0	1.3	11.4	5.6	1.7
Mallows (Peek Frean): see flavours						
Malt Bread	Sunblest SunMalt	268	8.3	56.8	2.4	N
Malt Loaf	Sunblest SunMalt	265	9.7	51.7	2.2	5.3
wholemeal	Allinson	259	10.6	48.2	2.6	6.8
Malt Vinegar	HP	4.0	0.4	0.6	n/a	nil

218

Malted Brown Bread	Hovis	233	8.8	43.0	2.2	4.8
Malted Brown Rolls	Hovis	254	10.4	44.6	3.2	4.4
Malted Food Drink (Horlicks): see Horlicks						
Malted Milk Creams	Boots	499	6.5	59.0	28.0	1.7
Maltesers	Mars	478	10.0	61.4	23.1	1.5
Maltlets, Horlicks	SmithKline Beecham	384	12.4	78.0	4.0	n/a
Malty Brown Bread	Nimble	240	9.2	43.7	2.5	5.2
Mandarin Oranges						
canned in juice		32.0	0.7	7.7	Tr	0.3
canned in syrup		52.0	0.5	14.4	Tr	0.2
Mandarin Style Special Rice	Heinz	141	5.7	22.4	3.2	0.8
Mandarin Yogurt, low calorie	Diet Ski	35.0	3.9	4.8	0.1	n/a
Mange-tout, raw		32.0	3.6	4.2	0.2	2.3
boiled		26.0	3.2	3.3	0.1	2.2
stir-fried		71.0	3.8	3.5	4.8	2.4
Mango & Apple Fruit Chutney	Sharwood	162	0.2	41.3	0.2	1.1

All amounts given per 100g/100ml unless otherwise stated

Product	Brand	Calories kcal	Protein (g)	Carbo-hydrate (g)	Fat (g)	Dietary Fibre (g)
Mango & Ginger Chutney	Sharwood	221	0.3	59.0	0.2	1.1
Mango Chutney, oily	Burgess	285	0.4	49.5	10.9	0.9
Green Label	Sharwood	241	0.3	58.6	Tr	0.8
	Sharwood	219	0.3	57.8	0.2	0.9
Mango Pickle	Sharwood	70.0	2.2	7.3	3.5	6.0
Mangoes *ripe, raw, flesh only*		57.0	0.7	14.1	0.2	2.6
canned in syrup		77.0	0.3	20.3	Tr	0.7
Mango/Pineapple in Light Syrup	Del Monte	63.0	0.6	15.9	Tr	n/a
Manor House Cake	Mr Kipling	425	5.2	54.0	22.4	n/a
Maple Flavour Pouring Syrup	Lyle's	284	Tr	76.0	nil	nil
Maple Walnut Ice Cream	Wall's Carte D'Or	150	2.5	14.0	10.0	n/a
Margarine (see also brands) average		739	0.2	1.0	81.6	nil
Marie Biscuits	Crawfords	470	6.7	74.2	15.7	2.3
	Peek Frean	442	6.6	71.8	14.3	2.1

Marmalade (see also flavours)						
	Applefords	261		69.5	nil	0.6
diabetic	Dietade	114	0.1	20.5	Tr	n/a
fine cut, diabetic	Boots	249	0.1	66.3	n/a	n/a
thick cut, diabetic	Boots	151	0.2	62.0	nil	1.6
		149	0.2	61.0	nil	1.7
Marmite		172	39.7	1.8	0.7	nil
Marrow						
raw, flesh only		12.0	0.5	2.2	0.2	0.5
boiled		9.0	0.4	1.6	0.2	0.6
Marrowfat Peas, canned		100	6.9	17.5	0.8	4.1
Mars Bar	Mars	432	5.6	68.6	16.9	1.2
Mars Milk	Mars	99.0	3.8	17.7	1.9	0.2
Marzipan, homemade		461	10.4	50.2	25.8	3.3
retail		404	5.3	67.6	14.4	1.9
Matchmakers						
coffee	Rowntree Mackintosh	476	4.1	68.4	22.6	n/a
mint	Rowntree Mackintosh	480	4.4	72.3	21.3	n/a

All amounts given per 100g/100ml unless otherwise stated

Product	Brand	Calories kcal	Protein (g)	Carbohydrate (g)	Fat (g)	Dietary Fibre (g)
orange	Rowntree Mackintosh	478	4.4	71.6	21.3	n/a
Mature Cheddar Cheese Spread, low fat	St Ivel Shape	162	12.6	6.0	9.9	n/a
Mature Cheddar Pasta Choice Dry Mix, as sold	Crosse & Blackwell	437	19.8	55.8	15.0	0.3
Mature Cheddar Sauce Mix, dry, as sold	Crosse & Blackwell Bonne Cuisine	480	21.0	34.5	28.7	0.8
Mature Cheese Wedge	St Ivel Shape	260	29.3	0.1	15.8	n/a
Matzos (Rakusen)	Rakusen	347	9.5	80.0	1.0	3.0
Matzos (Rakusen): see flavours						
Max the Lion Bars, each						
banana choc	Wall's	125	2.5	16.0	6.0	n/a
caramel choc	Wall's	125	2.5	16.0	6.0	n/a
Mayonnaise (see also flavours)						
	Heinz	691	1.1	1.7	75.6	nil
	HP	532	1.0	5.9	56.0	nil
		763	1.4	1.2	83.6	nil

reduced calorie	Boots Shapers	383	0.7	15.0	36.0	0.1
	Delight	53.0	0.1	1.2	5.3	n/a
	Heinz Weight Watchers	262	1.1	8.1	25.0	Tr
	Hellmanns	293	0.4	2.1	29.5	n/a
Meat Deluxe Pizza Slice	McCain Pizza Pantry	194	9.6	27.3	5.9	n/a
Meat Paste		173	15.2	3.0	11.2	0.1
Meatballs						
& beans & pasta	Campbell's	109	6.5	16.0	2.3	0.2
in beef gravy	Campbell's	90.0	4.7	12.9	2.3	0.3
in onion gravy	Campbell's	81.0	6.0	5.7	4.0	0.1
in tomato sauce	Campbell's	87.0	6.0	7.2	4.0	0.3
	Campbell's	87.0	6.0	7.2	4.0	0.2
Meatless Savoury Cuts	Granose	88.0	15.9	5.6	0.6	0.2
Mediterranean Fried Savoury Rice	Batchelors	368	9.5	67.4	8.6	n/a
Mediterranean Tomato Soup	Baxters	30.0	1.1	6.3	0.3	0.6
	Heinz Weight					

All amounts given per 100g/100ml unless otherwise stated

Product	Brand	Calories kcal	Protein (g)	Carbohydrate (g)	Fat (g)	Dietary Fibre (g)
Medium Curry Paste	Watchers	24.0	0.6	4.1	0.6	1.0
Medium Egg Noodles	Sharwood	247	4.7	5.8	22.7	8.6
Medium Fat Soft Cheese	Sharwood	332	10.8	70.1	1.8	2.9
Mega King Cone		179	9.2	3.1	14.5	nil
mint	Lyons Maid	367	6.2	46.4	18.7	n/a
	Lyons Maid	367	6.2	46.4	18.7	n/a
Mello Reduced Fat Spread	Vitalite	540	0.3	1.0	60.0	nil
Melon, flesh only						
Cantaloupe-type		19.0	0.6	4.2	0.1	1.0
Galia		24.0	0.5	5.6	0.1	0.4
Honeydew		28.0	0.6	6.6	0.1	0.6
Watermelon		31.0	0.5	7.1	0.3	0.1
Melon & Walnut Real Fruit						
Le Yogurt, stirred, low fat	Chambourcy	102	5.3	16.4	1.7	0.1
Melon Yogurt, low calorie	Diet Ski	35.0	3.9	4.8	0.2	n/a
MenuMaster Meals (Birds Eye): *see flavours*						
Meringue		379	5.3	95.4	Tr	nil

224

Mexican Bean Salad	Batchelors	133	8.1	21.2	1.7	n/a
Mexican Bean Stew	Granose	130	5.5	12.0	6.0	1.3
Mexican Chilli Cook-In-Sauce	Homepride	59.0	1.4	11.5	n/a	n/a
Mexican Chilli Cook In The Pot Microwave Mix, as sold	Crosse & Blackwell	328	13.1	43.5	11.3	5.3
Mexican Chilli Sauce						
mild	Homepride	61.0	1.4	11.7	n/a	n/a
medium	Homepride	59.0	1.4	11.8	n/a	n/a
hot	Homepride	59.0	1.2	11.9	n/a	n/a
extra hot	Homepride	59.0	1.2	11.4	n/a	n/a
Mexican Corn Roast	Granose	440	19.5	46.5	19.5	n/a
Mexican Cottage Cheese	St Ivel Shape	69.0	11.8	4.7	0.5	n/a
Mexican Salsa	Burgess	133	0.7	30.5	0.7	0.2
Mexicorn	Green Giant	72.0	n/a	n/a	0.2	n/a
frozen	Green Giant	87.0	n/a	n/a	0.8	n/a

Micro Chips: *see Chips, micro*

Microchef Meals & Snacks (Batchelors): *see flavours*

All amounts given per 100g/100ml unless otherwise stated

Product	Brand	Calories kcal	Protein (g)	Carbo-hydrate (g)	Fat (g)	Dietary Fibre (g)
Microwave Crumble Mix, as sold	Homepride	471	7.0	74.0	16.0	n/a
Mighty Bites	Ross	167	2.3	23.6	8.1	2.4
Mighty Muffins, each	Allied Bakeries	168	6.5	32.3	1.4	2.1
Mighty Munchers, each	Allied Bakeries	193	7.0	32.4	4.0	1.8
Mighty White Bread	Allied Bakeries	227	7.7	45.6	1.5	3.1
Mild Beer: see Beer						
Mild Cheese Rice Choice, as sold	Crosse & Blackwell	372	10.6	70.6	5.3	2.1
Mild Cheese Wedge	St Ivel Shape	262	29.1	0.2	16.1	n/a
Mild Curry Beanfeast	Batchelors	356	22.2	57.2	5.9	n/a
Mild Curry Paste	Sharwood	356	4.8	4.8	35.3	7.1
Mild Curry Rice Choice, as sold	Crosse & Blackwell	360	7.9	72.0	4.5	3.5
Mild Curry Savoury Rice	Batchelors	328	7.1	74.5	2.3	n/a
Mild Curry Supernoodles	Batchelors	474	7.4	56.2	26.0	n/a

Mild Kashmiri Curry Sauce, dry, as sold	Crosse & Blackwell Bonne Cuisine	379	12.8	52.0	13.3	3.4
Mild Mustard Pickle	Heinz Ploughman's	125	2.0	27.1	1.0	1.2
Mild Vegetable Curry	Sharwood	66.0	1.5	4.9	4.5	1.0
Milk (see also products, e.g. condensed, soya, etc)						
semi-skimmed, average		46.0	3.3	5.0	1.6	nil
skimmed, average		33.0	3.3	5.0	0.1	nil
whole, average		66.0	3.2	4.8	3.9	nil
Milk Chocolate	Nestlé	529	8.4	59.4	30.3	Tr
	Boots	520	7.4	60.3	29.5	n/a
diabetic		458	7.0	56.0	32.0	0.9
Milk Chocolate Bounty	Mars	471	4.6	56.4	26.8	3.8
Milk Chocolate Coated Sandwich Wafers, diabetic	Boots	523	11.0	50.0	31.0	2.8
Milk Chocolate Yorkie	Rowntree Mackintosh	510	7.5	57.5	29.4	n/a
Milk Club Biscuits	Jacob's	506	5.7	62.7	27.5	0.8

All amounts given per 100g/100ml unless otherwise stated

Product	Brand	Calories kcal	Protein (g)	Carbo-hydrate (g)	Fat (g)	Dietary Fibre (g)
Milk Coated Mallows	Peek Frean	457	4.5	69.8	19.7	0.5
Milk Pudding made with whole milk		129	3.9	19.9	4.3	0.1
made with semi-skimmed milk		93.0	4.0	20.1	0.2	0.1
Milk Tray	Cadbury	465	4.8	66.0	22.2	n/a
Milky Bar	Rowntree Mackintosh	545	8.0	58.0	33.0	n/a
Milky Bar Buttons	Rowntree Mackintosh	540	8.4	59.0	32.0	n/a
Milky Way	Mars	430	4.4	72.9	15.5	1.2
Millionaires Shortbread	California Cake & Cookie Co.	383	6.9	58.0	25.1	n/a
Milquik Powder, made up, per pint	St Ivel	200	20.7	30.1	0.7	n/a
Mince & Onion Beanfeast	Batchelors	346	29.4	48.7	5.0	n/a
Mince Bolognese	Tyne Brand	122	10.2	4.7	7.0	n/a
Mince Pies, each	Mr Kipling	207	2.2	33.7	8.1	n/a

Minced Beef: see Beef

Minced Beef & Onion Pastie	Ross	293	6.3	23.5	19.8	1.0
Minced Beef & Onion Pie						
canned	Tyne Brand	155	5.9	11.0	10.0	n/a
Golden Choice	Ross	295	6.6	24.6	19.4	1.0
Hungryman	Ross	249	6.4	20.7	16.0	0.9
Minced Beef Savoury Pancakes	Findus	161	7.2	23.0	4.5	1.0
Minced Beef with Vegetables & Gravy, per pack	Birds Eye MenuMaster	120	13.0	7.5	4.5	n/a
Minced Beef with Vegetables & Mashed Potato, per pack	Birds Eye MenuMaster	275	15.0	29.0	12.0	n/a
Mincemeat		274	0.6	62.1	4.3	1.3
Minestrone Soup						
canned	Baxters	30.0	1.3	6.0	0.2	1.0
	Heinz	31.0	1.4	4.5	0.8	0.5
canned, low calorie	Heinz Weight Watchers	18.0	1.0	2.8	0.3	0.4
dried, as sold		298	10.1	47.6	8.8	N

All amounts given per 100g/100ml unless otherwise stated

Product	Brand	Calories kcal	Protein (g)	Carbohydrate (g)	Fat (g)	Dietary Fibre (g)
dried, as served		23.0	0.8	3.7	8.8	N
Minestrone Soup with Croutons	Boots Shapers	346	56.0	56.0	8.2	2.9
Mini Milk Ice Cream, all varieties, each	Wall's	35.0	1.0	6.0	1.0	n/a
Minstrels, Galaxy	Mars	474	6.0	69.5	21.0	1.0
Mint Assortment	Cravens	395	0.3	88.8	5.6	Tr
Mint Choc Chip Bar, each	Wall's	196	2.2	18.4	13.2	n/a
Mint Choc Chip Dairy Ice Cream	Lyons Maid Napoli	112	1.9	15.0	5.0	n/a
Mint Choc Ice Cream	Wall's Gino Ginelli Tubs	120	1.5	15.0	6.0	n/a
Mint Club Biscuits	Jacob's	500	4.3	63.3	27.3	0.8
Mint Creams, each	Trebor Bassett	32.0	n/a	8.4	n/a	n/a
Mint Crisp, each	Lyons Maid	179	2.3	20.1	10.5	n/a
Mint Flavour Milk Chocolate Coated Sandwich Wafers,						

			519	10.0	20.0	31.0	2.3
diabetic		Boots					
Mint Humbugs diabetic	Cravens	Boots	400	0.7	88.5	6.0	nil
	Boots		262	0.6	92.0	4.3	Tr
Mint Imperials	Trebor Bassett		392	0.3	98.0	0.2	nil
Mint Jelly	Baxters		251	Tr	67.0	Tr	1.7
	Burgess		174	0.3	43.1	nil	Tr
	Colman's		263	0.1	n/a	Tr	Tr
Mint Leaves	Cadbury		450	3.2	67.8	20.2	n/a
Mint Sauce	Baxters		110	0.9	28.1	0.2	Tr
	Burgess		76.0	1.0	14.5	nil	0.9
	HP		156	2.1	26.1	1.7	n/a
fresh garden	Colman's		99.0	0.8	n/a	Tr	Tr
Mint Toffees each	Itona		360	0.6	67.0	11.0	n/a
	Trebor Bassett		31.0	n/a	4.5	1.4	n/a
Mint Viennetta	Wall's		130	2.0	14.0	8.0	n/a
Mint YoYo	McVitie's		523	4.7	63.9	27.7	0.8
Minties	Rowntree Mackintosh		385	0.5	93.0	3.8	n/a

All amounts given per 100g/100ml unless otherwise stated

Product	Brand	Calories kcal	Protein (g)	Carbo-hydrate (g)	Fat (g)	Dietary Fibre (g)
Mintoes	Cravens	408	Tr	84.4	9.1	nil
Mintola	Rowntree Mackintosh	436	1.9	75.1	16.3	n/a
Mints: see individual types or flavours						
Minty Easter Egg, each	Rowntree Mackintosh	157	1.0	29.6	4.7	n/a
Miracle Whip Dressing	Kraft	440	1.0	12.0	43.0	n/a
Miso		203	13.3	23.5	6.2	N
Mississippi Mud Pie	California cake & Cookie Co.	431	4.25	53.8	23.8	2.3
Mr Brain's Meals (Kraft): see flavours						
Mister Men Lollies, each						
dairy strawberry	Lyons Maid	49.0	1.2	8.6	1.3	n/a
dairy vanilla	Lyons Maid	50.0	1.2	8.8	1.4	n/a
orange	Lyons Maid	29.0	nil	7.0	nil	n/a
strawberry	Lyons Maid	29.0	nil	7.0	nil	n/a
Mr Softee Soft Ice Cream	Lyons Maid	140	3.0	20.2	5.8	n/a

cornish dairy	Lyons Maid	141	3.0	20.2	5.8	n/a
Mivvis (Lyons Maid): *see flavours*						
Mixed Bean Salad, canned	Heinz	175	3.6	16.6	10.5	4.3
Mixed Cheese Salad, per pack	Boots	265	n/a	n/a	n/a	n/a
Mixed Fruit, dried		227	3.6	52.9	1.6	2.2
Mixed Fruit Bar, each	Granose	169	23.	24.0	7.0	6.0
Mixed Fruit Jam	Dietade	249	0.2	66.1	n/a	n/a
Mixed Fruit Sponge Pudding	Heinz	310	3.6	46.9	12.0	2.5
Mixed Nuts		607	22.9	7.9	54.1	6.0
Mixed Peel		231	0.3	59.1	0.9	4.8
Mixed Peppers	Ross	19.0	1.0	4.9	0.2	1.5
dried	Whitworths	212	12.3	30.1	5.5	12.3
Mixed Peppers Rice Choice, as sold	Crosse & Blackwell	368	9.0.	74.7	3.7	3.3
Mixed Vegetables						
frozen, boiled		42.0	3.3	6.6	0.5	N
canned		38.0	1.9	6.1	0.8	1.7
stir fry type, frozen, fried in oil		64.0	2.0	6.4	3.6	N

All amounts given per 100g/100ml unless otherwise stated

Product	Brand	Calories kcal	Protein (g)	Carbo-hydrate (g)	Fat (g)	Dietary Fibre (g)
Mock Duck	Granose	194	21.4	13.7	4.0	n/a
Moghlai Chicken Korma Microwave Meal	Sharwood	162	7.0	17.0	7.8	1.4
Monkey Nuts: see Peanuts						
Mooli: see Radish, white						
Moonshine	Libby	48.0	Tr	12.0	Tr	nil
Morello Cherry Jam, reduced sugar	Heinz Weight Watchers	125	0.4	33.0	Tr	0.9
Morello Cherry Ice Cream	Wall's Carte D'Or	115	2.0	18.0	4.5	n/a
Mountain Berries Yogurt	Alpine Ski	93.0	5.0	17.9	0.7	n/a
Moussaka		184	9.1	7.0	13.6	0.9
	Findus Lean Cuisine	76.0	5.2	8.5	2.2	0.9
	Findus Dinner Supreme	122	7.1	10.9	5.9	0.6
Moussaka Cook In The Pot Dry Mix, as sold	Crosse & Blackwell	321	14.0	45.4	9.3	5.7

Mousse: see flavours

Muesli (see also flavours)

Swiss style		363	9.8	72.2	5.9	6.4
with no added sugar		366	10.5	67.1	7.8	7.6
Muesli Cookie	California Cake & Cookie Co.	400	3.8	54.8	19.2	4.9
Muesli Crispbread	Kavli	285	11.3	60.5	1.4	19.4
Muesli Fritters	Granose	145	3.9	13.8	8.5	n/a
Muesli Yogurt	St Ivel Shape	47.0	4.9	6.1	0.4	n/a
Muffins	Sunblest	214	7.6	42.9	1.3	1.7
with cheese	Sunblest	221	8.4	40.2	2.9	1.4
Mulligatawny Soup	Heinz Spicy Soups	57.0	1.7	5.9	3.0	0.2
Munchies	Rowntree Mackintosh	472	5.6	65.8	22.5	n/a
Munchmallows	McVitie's	448	5.3	70.0	16.5	1.1
Mung beans, boiled		91.0	7.6	15.3	0.4	4.8

All amounts given per 100g/100ml unless otherwise stated

235

Product	Brand	Calories kcal	Protein (g)	Carbo-hydrate (g)	Fat (g)	Dietary Fibre (g)
Mung Beansprouts: see Beansprouts						
Murray Mints	Trebor Basset	410	nil	92.0	5.2	nil
Mushroom A La Creme Pasta Choice Dry Mix, as sold	Crosse & Blackwell	402	15.9	63.6	9.3	0.7
Mushroom & Bacon Toast Topper	Heinz	87.0	6.4	6.7	3.8	0.5
Mushroom & Garlic Croisanti	McVitie's	319	8.4	30.9	18.6	1.3
Mushroom & Wine Pasta & Sauce	Batchelors	352	13.0	71.4	3.6	n/a
Mushroom Cream Pasta Sauce, dry, as sold	Buitoni	388	12.3	50.3	15.3	2.8
Mushroom Feasts, each	Birds Eye	98.0	2.0	12.0	5.0	n/a
Mushroom Ketchup	Burgess	27.0	0.4	5.5	0.1	Tr
Mushroom Pasta Sauce	Dolmio	164	2.6	4.5	15.1	n/a
Mushroom Pate per tub	Tartex	241	6.5	11.0	19.0	0.3
	Vessen	120	2.9	5.8	8.1	0.1

	Brand					
Mushroom Rice Choice, as sold	Crosse & Blackwell	369	9.2	73.5	4.2	2.5
Mushroom Sauce Mix, as sold	Colman's	367	14.0	n/a	9.7	n/a
Mushroom Savoury Rice	Batchelors	339	8.3	76.2	2.2	n/a
Mushroom Soup, instant, as sold	Boots Shapers	314	6.5	54.0	8.0	2.6
Mushrooms						
common, raw		13.0	1.8	0.4	0.5	1.1
common, boiled		11.0	1.8	0.4	0.3	1.1
common, fried in oil		157	2.4	0.3	16.2	1.5
common, canned		12.0	2.1	Tr	0.4	1.3
Chinese, dried, raw		284	10.0	59.9	1.8	N
oyster, raw		8.0	1.6	Tr	0.2	N
shiitake, dried, raw		296	9.6	63.9	1.0	N
shiitake, cooked		55.0	1.6	12.3	0.2	N
straw, canned, drained		15.0	2.1	1.2	0.2	N
Mushrooms Vegetarian Spread	Granose	231	10.1	10.0	16.8	n/a
Mushy Peas, canned		81.0	5.8	13.8	0.7	1.8

All amounts given per 100g/100ml unless otherwise stated

Product	Brand	Calories kcal	Protein (g)	Carbo-hydrate (g)	Fat (g)	Dietary Fibre (g)
Mussels, boiled		87.0	17.2	Tr	2.0	nil
Mustard *(see also flavours)*						
smooth		139	7.1	9.7	8.2	N
wholegrain		140	8.2	4.2	10.2	4.9
Mustard & Onion Mello 'n' Mild	Colman's	143	3.9	n/a	4.0	n/a
Mustard Dip, per pack	Kavli	350	6.9	6.0	33.3	n/a

Product	Brand	Calories kcal	Protein (g)	Carbo-hydrate (g)	Fat (g)	Dietary Fibre (g)
Naan Bread		336	8.9	50.1	12.5	1.9
Nachips	Old El Paso	463	n/a	n/a	n/a	n/a

Food	Brand					
Napoletana Pasta Sauce						
chilled	Dolmio	36.0	1.5	6.7	0.5	n/a
with red wine (jar)	Dolmio	30.0	0.8	6.6	Tr	n/a
with vegetables (jar)	Dolmio	44.0	0.9	5.4	2.1	1.3
Napolitan Pasta Choice Dry Mix, as sold	Crosse & Blackwell	371	11.3	72.4	4.0	1.3
Natural Cottage Cheese	Eden Vale	97.0	13.7	1.6	4.0	n/a
diet	St Ivel Shape	71.0	13.4	3.5	0.5	n/a
	Eden Vale Bodyline	83.0	13.0	3.6	1.9	n/a
Natural Country Bran	Jordans	190	15.0	27.0	4.0	4.0
Natural Goats Milk Yogurt	Holland & Barrett	65.0	3.8	2.9	4.8	n/a
Natural Harvest Mushy Peas, canned	Batchelors	84.0	5.7	15.2	0.5	n/a
Natural Harvest Processed Peas, canned	Batchelors	78.0	6.5	13.0	0.4	n/a
Natural Soft Cheese, low fat	St Ivel Shape	132	11.7	2.7	8.4	n/a
Natural Wheatgerm	Jordans	337	26.0	49.0	8.0	12.0

All amounts given per 100g/100ml unless otherwise stated

Product	Brand	Calories kcal	Protein (g)	Carbohydrate (g)	Fat (g)	Dietary Fibre (g)
Natural Yogurt	Eden Vale	71.0	6.8	9.4	1.0	n/a
	St Ivel	60.0	5.8	6.7	1.5	n/a
Greek Style	Holland & Barrett	142	5.3	7.7	10.0	nil
low fat	Holland & Barrett	65.0	5.7	8.3	1.0	nil
Neapolitan Ice Cream	Lyons Maid Wall's Gino Ginelli	85.0	1.8	10.5	4.0	n/a
reduced fat	Heinz Weight Watchers	85.0	1.5	11.0	4.0	n/a
		68.0	1.7	7.4	2.8	Tr
Neapolitan Wafers	Peek Frean	503	4.7	61.0	28.4	1.2
Nectarine & Tangerine Yogurt	St Ivel Shape	43	5.1	5.9	0.1	n/a
Nectarine Yogurt, bio stirred	Ski	113	5.8	16.7	3.0	n/a
Nectarines, flesh & skin		40.0	1.4	9.0	0.1	1.2
Neeps (England): see Swede						
Neeps (Scotland): see Turnip						

Nesquik (Nestlé): *see flavours*

New Potatoes: *see Potatoes, new*

Nibblers, frozen	Green Giant	100	n/a	n/a	n/a	1.0	n/a
Niblets	Green Giant	70.0	n/a	20.0	n/a	nil	n/a
no added salt/sugar	Green Giant	69.0	n/a	73.3	n/a	0.2	n/a
Nice Biscuits	Boots	476	6.5	73.3	n/a	n/a	3.2
	Peek Frean	434	6.1	n/a	n/a	14.9	2.3
Nice Creams	Peek Frean	484	5.0	71.0	n/a	21.8	2.5
Nobbly Bobbly Mivvi, each	Lyons Maid	268	38.6	2.2	n/a	12.7	n/a
Non-dairy Ice Cream: *see Ice Cream*							
Noodle Doodles Spaghetti Shapes in Tomato Sauce	Heinz	63.0	1.5	13.5	n/a	0.3	0.7
Noodles, egg, boiled		62.0	2.2	13.0	n/a	0.5	0.6
North Atlantic Peeled Prawns	Young's	70.0	16.4	nil	n/a	0.5	n/a
Northumbrian Teacakes	Mothers Pride	282	8.5	49.8	n/a	5.3	2.5
Number 7 Cider	Bulmer	33.0	n/a	n/a	n/a	n/a	n/a
Nut & Chocolate Slices, each	Mr Kipling	150	3.6	13.6	n/a	9.4	n/a

All amounts given per 100g/100ml unless otherwise stated

Product	Brand	Calories kcal	Protein (g)	Carbo-hydrate (g)	Fat (g)	Dietary Fibre (g)
Nut & Sesame Burgers	Granose	329	12.0	29.0	18.0	n/a
Nut Crisp, per standard bar	Cadbury	210	2.8	24.1	11.8	n/a
Nut Fruit Snack Bar, each	Granose	95.0	2.0	16.2	2.5	2.2
Nut Krisps	Lyons	511	5.5	59.9	29.4	0.9
Nut Loaf	Granose	176	18.9	4.9	9.1	3.4
Nut Meringue Gateau	McVitie's	401	2.7	35.2	27.8	0.2
Nut Roast	Granose	488	35.0	20.2	27.8	n/a
Nutbrawn	Granose	212	8.3	13.2	14.4	n/a
Nuts & Raisins, per pack	Golden Wonder	217	6.6	14.4	15.2	n/a
Nuttolene	Granose	298	13.1	11.0	22.7	4.2
Nutty Crunchy Cereal	Holland & Barrett	361	10.5	60.0	12.0	12.0
Nutty Toffee Dairy Ice Cream	Lyons Maid Napoli	99.0	2.4	12.2	3.5	n/a

Oat & Wheat Bran	Weetabix	328	11.5	60.5	4.4	17.8
Oat Crispy Crunch	Mornflake	378	12.9	60.0	13.0	6.9
Oat Fingers, each	Paterson's	45.0	n/a	n/a	1.9	n/a
Oat Krunchies	Quaker	383	10.7	71.7	7.3	6.5
Oatbran	Jordans	340	17.0	65.0	9.0	15.0
	Mornflake	383	16.2	59.0	8.0	18.5
Oatbran Hearts	Jordans	364	11.4	57.6	11.4	13.5
with raisins & sliced apple	Jordans	368	10.2	53.4	14.1	12.2
Oatcakes		441	10.0	63.0	18.3	N
Oatmeal Bread	Crofters Kitchen	234	8.1	41.6	3.9	3.7
Ocean Pie	Ross Recipe Meal	117	6.6	9.5	6.0	0.4

All amounts given per 100g/100ml unless otherwise stated

Product	Brand	Calories kcal	Protein (g)	Carbo-hydrate (g)	Fat (g)	Dietary Fibre (g)
Oil-Free French dressing	Waistline	11.0	0.7	0.3	0.2	0.1
Oil-Free Vinaigrette	Waistline	13.0	0.7	0.7	0.2	0.2
Okra (gumbo, lady's fingers)						
boiled		28.0	2.5	2.7	0.9	3.6
stir-fried		269	4.3	4.4	26.1	6.3
canned, drained		21.0	1.4	2.5	0.7	2.6
Old Fashioned Jumbo Oats	Mornflake	370	12.0	65.0	8.7	7.0
Old Jamaica	Cadbury	480	6.5	59.3	26.0	n/a
Olde English Toasting Muffins	Mothers Pride	225	11.2	39.5	1.9	2.9
Olive Oil						
pure	Napolina	899	Tr	nil	99.9	nil
extra virgin	Napolina	900	n/a	nil	100	nil
		900	n/a	nil	100	nil
Olives, pitted, in brine		103	0.9	Tr	11.0	2.9
Olives Vegetarian Spread	Granose	247	10.4	8.9	18.8	n/a
Omelette, plain		191	10.9	Tr	16.4	nil
cheese		266	15.9	Tr	22.6	nil

244

100% Beefburgers, each	Birds Eye Steakhouse	120	9.0	9.0	0.5	9.0	n/a
Onion & Cheddar Cottage Cheese	St Ivel Shape	91.0	11.9	3.1	4.2	3.1	n/a
Onion & Chive Cottage Cheese diet	Eden Vale Eden Vale Bodyline	93.0 81.0	13.0 12.7	3.9 1.9	1.7 3.6	3.9 1.9	n/a n/a
Onion & Chive Dip	Burgess	472	2.0	45.8	11.7	45.8	0.4
Onion & Chive Dressing	Burgess	488	1.7	48.5	10.1	48.5	0.1
Onion Bhajia Mix	Sharwood	330	10.8	3.6	61.0	3.6	5.1
Onion Bhajis	Ross	165	6.8	6.0	24.7	6.0	3.7
Onion, Chives & Dill Cottage Cheese	St Ivel Shape	66.0	12.0	0.4	3.7	0.4	n/a
Onion Relish	Branston	125	0.7	0.3	31.7	0.3	1.0
Onion Ringers	Ross	243	3.9	12.5	31.2	12.5	2.4
Onion Sauce made with whole milk		99.0	2.8	6.5	8.3	6.5	0.4

All amounts given per 100g/100ml unless otherwise stated

Product	Brand	Calories kcal	Protein (g)	Carbohydrate (g)	Fat (g)	Dietary Fibre (g)
made with semi-skimmed milk		86.0	2.9	8.4	5.0	0.4
Onions						
raw		36.0	1.2	7.9	0.2	1.4
baked		103	3.5	22.3	0.6	3.9
boiled		17.0	0.6	3.7	0.1	0.7
fried in oil		164	2.3	14.1	11.2	3.1
dried, raw		313	10.2	68.6	1.7	12.1
pickled, drained		24.0	0.9	4.9	0.2	1.2
cocktail/silverskin, drained		15.0	0.6	3.1	0.1	N
Onions & Garlic Ragu	Brooke Bond	80.0	1.8	12.6	2.8	n/a
Opal Fruits	Mars	389	0.3	85.3	7.6	n/a
Orange & Almond Pudding	McVitie's	378	4.2	44.2	21.1	1.4
Orange & Carob Crunchy Bar	Jordans	411	9.0	51.9	20.1	5.4
Orange & Cream Mivvi, each	Lyons Maid	87.0	1.1	14.2	2.8	n/a
Orange & Lemon Gateau	McVitie's	292	2.4	31.7	17.5	0.4
Orange & Lemon Slices, diabetic	Boots	234	7.9	81.0	0.3	nil

Orange & Lychee Tropical Yogurt	St Ivel Shape	43.0	4.7	5.7	0.2	n/a
Orange & Oat Mini Cookies	Boots	486	5.3	64.0	25.0	2.9
Orange & Pineapple Drink low calorie	Quosh	32.0	n/a	8.4	n/a	n/a
sparkling	Boots Shapers	21.0	0.3	5.2	nil	nil
sparkling, low calorie	Tango	44.0	n/a	11.6	n/a	n/a
	Diet Tango	2.0	n/a	0.6	n/a	n/a
Orange & Pineapple Fruit Juice	Del Monte	42.0	0.5	10.8	Tr	n/a
Orange & Raisin Crunch 'n' Slim	Crookes Healthcare	405	10.5	55.0	17.6	11.2
Orange & Raspberry Drink	Boots Shapers	20.0	n/a	n/a	Tr	nil
Orange & Sherry Chinese Spare Rib Sauce	Sharwood	181	3.0	37.7	2.2	1.8
Orange & Walnut Crunchy	Mornflake	412	10.6	64.9	12.9	15.0
Orange Apple Passionfruit Juice	Del Monte	42.0	0.5	11.2	0.1	n/a

All amounts given per 100g/100ml unless otherwise stated

Product	Brand	Calories kcal	Protein (g)	Carbo-hydrate (g)	Fat (g)	Dietary Fibre (g)
Orange Barley Crush, sparkling (Lucozade): see Lucozade						
Orange Barley Water	Robinsons	22.0	Tr	n/a	Tr	n/a
Orange 'C'	Libby	37.0	0.1	9.1	Tr	0.1
Orange Carob Coated Fruit Bar	Granose	169	2.7	31.8	3.5	2.3
Orange Citrus Lunchbar	Boots Shapers	409	8.3	49.0	20.0	n/a
Orange Club Biscuits	Jacob's	510	5.5	62.3	28.2	0.7
Orange Coated Mallows	Peek Frean	456	4.5	69.5	19.7	0.5
Orange Cream, per bar	Cadbury	210	1.6	37.1	7.2	n/a
Orange Cream Biscuits	Cadbury	508	5.4	65.7	26.6	n/a
Orange Crunchies, diabetic	Boots	444	5.5	59.0	24.0	4.4
Orange Drink, undiluted		107	Tr	28.5	nil	nil
low calorie	Quosh	5.0	n/a	0.9	n/a	n/a
original, ready to drink	Robinsons	31.0	Tr	n/a	n/a	n/a
sparkling	Jusoda	31.0	n/a	n/a	n/a	n/a
	St Clements	43.0	n/a	n/a	n/a	n/a
	Tango	46.0	n/a	12.3	n/a	n/a

sparkling, low calorie	Diet Jusoda	31.0	n/a	n/a	n/a	n/a	n/a
	Diet Tango	3.0	n/a	0.8	0.2	n/a	n/a
Orange Flavour Jelly Crystals	Dietade	7.0	1.5	0.2	n/a	n/a	n/a
Orange Flavour Milk Chocolate, diabetic	Boots	458	10.0	48.5	32.0	32.0	4.2
Orange Flavour Milk Chocolate Coated Sandwich Wafers, diabetic	Boots	514	10.0	48.5	32.0	32.0	4.2
Orange Flavour Sandwich Wafers, diabetic	Boots	506	11.0	51.0	30.0	30.0	2.7
Orange Fruit Drink, undiluted	Baby Ribena	316	0.5	84.0	n/a	n/a	n/a
Orange Fruit Juice	Del Monte	39.0	0.6	9.7	Tr	Tr	n/a
Orange Fruitie, each	Wall's	55.0	Tr	15.0	Tr	Tr	n/a
Orange Instant Chocolate Drink	Boots Shapers	367	17.0	57.0	9.5	9.5	4.5
Orange Jelly, ready to eat	Rowntree	78.0	Tr	19.6	Tr	Tr	0.6
Orange Juice, unsweetened		36.0	0.5	8.8	0.1	0.1	0.1

All amounts given per 100g/100ml unless otherwise stated

Product	Brand	Calories kcal	Protein (g)	Carbohydrate (g)	Fat (g)	Dietary Fibre (g)
Orange Krisps	Lyons	534	5.4	62.4	31.0	0.4
Orange, Lemon & Pineapple Whole Fruit Drink	Robinsons	20.0	Tr	n/a	Tr	n/a
Orange Maid Mivvi, each	Lyons Maid	45.0	Tr	11.0	nil	n/a
Orange Marmalade fine shred	Baxters	200	Tr	53.0	Tr	0.4
reduced sugar, thin cut	Heinz Weight Watchers	125	0.4	33.0	Tr	0.1
vintage	Baxters	200	Tr	53.0	Tr	0.8
Orange Mini Rolls, each	Cadbury	103	1.4	14.4	4.8	n/a
Orange Monster Mousse	St Ivel Fiendish Feet	57.0	2.1	9.4	1.5	n/a
Orange Peach Apricot Juice	Del Monte	39.0	0.6	9.7	Tr	n/a
Orange Sorbet Fromage Frais	St Ivel Shape	52.0	6.8	6.0	0.2	n/a
Orange Soya Dessert	Granose	94.0	1.3	14.6	3.8	n/a
Orange Squash undiluted	St Clements	135	0.2	32.0	0.1	n/a

light, undiluted low calorie	St Clements / Dietade	26.0 / 12.0	0.3 / n/a	4.4 / 2.4	0.1 / n/a	n/a / n/a
Orange Trembler	St Ivel Fiendish Feet	75.0	2.7	16.2	0.4	n/a
Orange Truffles	Rowntree Mackintosh	457	5.0	66.5	20.8	n/a
Orange Whole Fruit Drink	Robinsons	20.4	Tr	n/a	Tr	n/a
Orange Wholemeal Cake Mix, as sold	Granose	427	13.1	55.5	13.2	n/a
Orange Yogurt	St Ivel Real / Ski	83.0 / 88.0	4.9 / 5.0	13.6 / 16.4	1.1 / 0.7	n/a / n/a
Orange Yogurt Drink	Ski Cool	72.0	3.2	15.0	0.3	n/a
Orange YoYo	McVitie's	523	4.7	63.8	27.6	1.0
Orangeade	Corona	27.0	n/a	7.1	n/a	n/a
Orangeade Sparkles, each	Wall's	30.0	Tr	8.0	Tr	n/a
Oranges, flesh only		37.0	1.1	8.5	0.1	1.7
Orangina Sparkling Orange Juice	Bulmer	38.0	n/a	n/a	n/a	n/a

All amounts given per 100g/100ml unless otherwise stated

251

Product	Brand	Calories kcal	Protein (g)	Carbo-hydrate (g)	Fat (g)	Dietary Fibre (g)
Orbit Sugarfree Chewing Gum, all flavours	Wrigley	275	nil	2.4	nil	n/a
Orchards Fruit Pie	McVitie's	272	3.8	38.4	12.0	1.1
Oregano, fresh dried, ground		66.0 306	2.2 11.0	9.7 49.5	2.0 10.3	N N
Organic Cider Vinegar	Applefords	25.0	0.1	nil	nil	n/a
Organic Flour Bread	Allinson	218	9.3	39.3	2.6	6.5
Organic Grade Porridge Oats	Jordans	396	13.6	72.6	9.0	6.3
Organic Grade Wholewheat & Raisins	Jordans	292	9.0	65.5	1.2	6.5
Organic Oat Crunchy	Mornflake	370	10.0	52.0	11.0	10.0
Organic Oatcakes, each	Vessen	99.0	2.5	13.2	3.8	1.4
Organic Oats	Mornflake	376	12.0	72.0	9.0	7.0
Oriental Beef French Bread Pizza	Findus Lean Cuisine	174	10.5	23.5	4.2	1.3
Oriental Beef Stir Fry Cook	Crosse &

In The Pot Dry Mix, as sold	Blackwell	371	7.7	65.3	8.8	1.5
Oriental Casserole	Granose	89.0	1.0	12.0	4.0	n/a
Oriental Chicken	Batchelors Microchef Meal	83.0	6.0	12.9	1.2	n/a
Snack Pot	Boots Shapers	101	7.6	15.0	1.6	1.0
Oriental Chicken Stir Fry Cook In The Pot Dry Mix, as sold	Crosse & Blackwell	386	7.1	61.8	12.3	1.8
Oriental Mix	Ross	37.0	1.8	8.1	0.3	1.3
Original Beefburgers, each	Birds Eye Steakhouse	120	9.0	1.5	8.5	n/a
Original Carmelle Mix, made up, per serving	Homepride	151	5.0	22.0	5.5	n/a
Original Cheese Wedge	St Ivel Shape	259	27.1	0.5	16.5	n/a
Original Cheesecake Mix, made up, per serving	Homepride	218	3.0	22.5	12.5	n/a
Original Cider bottled	Bulmer	37.0	n/a	n/a	n/a	n/a

All amounts given per 100g/100ml unless otherwise stated

Product	Brand	Calories kcal	Protein (g)	Carbohydrate (g)	Fat (g)	Dietary Fibre (g)
draught	Bulmer	32.0	n/a	n/a	n/a	n/a
Original Crunchy Bar (Jordans): see flavours						
Original Crunchy Cereal with oatbran & apple	Jordans	360	9.3	59.0	9.8	7.4
with raisins & rippled almond	Jordans	359	9.0	59.6	10.2	7.1
with tropical fruits	Jordans	394	8.5	58.0	15.3	7.0
Original Dolmio Pasta Sauce	Dolmio	37.0	0.9	8.4	Tr	n/a
with mushrooms	Dolmio	36.0	0.9	7.9	Tr	n/a
with spicy peppers	Dolmio	36.0	0.9	8.2	Tr	n/a
original lite	Dolmio	24.0	0.8	5.2	Tr	n/a
Original Honey Oatbran Bar	Jordans	413	9.1	47.5	22.0	7.6
Original Mixed Vegetables, 1oz/28g	Birds Eye	13.0	1.0	2.5	Tr	n/a
Outline Dairy Spread, very low fat	Van Den Berghs	265	2.5	8.0	25.0	n/a
Ovaltine, powder		358	9.0	79.4	2.7	N
made up with whole milk		97.0	3.8	12.9	3.8	Tr

		79.0	3.9	13.0	1.7	Tr
made up with semi-skimmed milk		79.0	3.9	13.0	1.7	Tr
Oven Chips: see Chips, oven						
Oven Crispy Cod Steaks, each	Birds Eye	230	12.0	13.0	15.0	n/a
Oven Crispy Haddock Steaks, each	Birds Eye	230	12.0	5.0	15.0	n/a
Oven Crispy Fingers, each	Birds Eye	80.0	3.5	5.0	5.5	n/a
Oxo Beef Drink, as served	Brooke Bond	3.9	0.7	0.2	nil	n/a
Oxo Cubes, as sold	Brooke Bond	263	23.4	58.8	6.9	n/a
chicken	Brooke Bond	246	24.3	28.4	4.8	n/a
vegetable	Brooke Bond	245	10.6	46.1	3.3	n/a
Oxtail, stewed		243	30.5	nil	13.4	nil
Oxtail Soup canned	Crosse & Blackwell	34.0	2.0	5.1	0.6	0.2
	Heinz	44.0	2.3	6.0	1.2	0.1
	Campbell's	76.0	2.9	10.3	2.6	0.2
condensed, as sold		356	17.6	51.0	10.5	N
dried, as served		27.0	1.4	3.9	0.8	N

All amounts given per 100g/100ml unless otherwise stated

Product	Brand	Calories kcal	Protein (g)	Carbo-hydrate (g)	Fat (g)	Dietary Fibre (g)
Oyster Chinese Pouring Sauce	Sharwood	75.0	1.3	17.0	0.2	0.3

P

Product	Brand	Calories kcal	Protein (g)	Carbo-hydrate (g)	Fat (g)	Dietary Fibre (g)
Pacific Pilchards						
in brine	Armour	187	22.0	nil	11.0	n/a
in tomato sauce	Armour	126	19.0	1.0	5.0	n/a
Pacific Salmon Slices	Young's	130	25.1	n/a	3.3	n/a
Paella						
Fast Cook	Vesta	123	4.4	20.1	3.3	n/a
	Ross Recipe Meal	94.0	5.6	15.8	1.4	0.9
Paglia e Fieno	Dolmio	125	4.6	25.6	1.2	n/a

Pale Ale, bottled		32.0	0.3	2.0	Tr	nil
Palm Oil		899	Tr	nil	99.9	nil
Pancake Mix, made up, per serving as sold	Homepride Perfect	104	4.0	15.0	3.0	nil
	Whitworths	348	12.6	76.6	1.1	nil
Pancake Roll		217	6.6	20.9	12.5	N
Pancakes (see also flavours) savoury, made with whole milk		273	6.3	24.0	17.5	0.8
sweet, made with whole milk		301	5.9	35.0	16.2	0.8
Pancho Peanuts, each	Trebor Bassett	6.0	n/a	0.4	0.5	Tr
Pancho Raisins, each	Trebor Bassett	6.0	n/a	0.4	0.5	Tr
Panini Pizza, each	Birds Eye Gino Ginelli	300	12.0	28.0	16.0	n/a
Papaya, unripe, raw		27.0	0.9	5.5	0.1	1.5
Papaya/Pineapple in Light Syrup	Del Monte	64.0	0.6	16.3	Tr	n/a
Paradise Slices	Lyons	481	5.3	50.1	30.3	7.3

All amounts given per 100g/100ml unless otherwise stated

Product	Brand	Calories kcal	Protein (g)	Carbo-hydrate (g)	Fat (g)	Dietary Fibre (g)
Parfait Bar						
milk	Lyons Tetley	521	6.3	58.5	30.8	n/a
plain	Lyons Tetley	529	5.0	55.2	33.6	n/a
Parmesan Cheese	Napolina	452	39.4	Tr	32.7	nil
		480	46.0	Tr	37.0	n/a
Parmesan Pasta & Sauce	Batchelors	372	15.8	68.0	6.0	n/a
Parmesan Style Ragu	Brooke Bond	90.0	2.9	12.1	2.6	n/a
Parsley Sauce						
dry mix, as sold	Colman's	331	1.0	n/a	1.7	n/a
	Knorr	348	6.7	61.5	10.0	4.3
Pour Over	Knorr	73.0	2.2	8.1	3.8	Tr
Parsnip, boiled		66.0	1.6	12.9	1.2	4.7
Partridge, roast, meat only		212	36.7	nil	7.2	nil
Passanda Classic Curry Sauce, jar	Homepride	103	2.7	13.2	n/a	n/a
Passion Cake Mix, made up, per serving	Green's	375	4.0	42.0	23.0	n/a

Passionfruit, flesh & pips only		36.0	2.6	5.8	0.4	3.3
Passionfruit Fruit Snack Bar, each	Granose	87.0	0.7	18.0	1.2	2.5
Passionfruit Melba Sundae Yogurt	St Ivel Shape	43.0	4.9	5.6	0.1	n/a
Pasta						
egg, cooked, all shapes	Buitoni	132	5.2	24.4	1.5	1.3
standard, cooked, all shapes	Buitoni	129	4.8	25.9	0.7	1.2
Pasta Bolognese	Batchelors Microchef Meal	114	5.9	13.4	4.5	n/a
	Boots Shapers	74.0	4.7	10.0	2.0	1.3
Snack Pot	Boots Shapers	68.0	5.0	8.4	1.8	2.8
Pasta Carbonara Instant Pot Meal	Boots Shapers	387	12.0	64.0	11.0	n/a
Pasta Cheese & Vegetables	Dolmio Ready Meals	99.0	2.5	9.7	5.9	n/a
Pasta Choice (Crosse & Blackwell): see flavours						
Pasta Salad	Eden Vale	190	3.1	14.1	13.9	n/a
canned	Heinz	194	1.9	21.0	11.4	0.7

All amounts given per 100g/100ml unless otherwise stated

Product	Brand	Calories kcal	Protein (g)	Carbo-hydrate (g)	Fat (g)	Dietary Fibre (g)
Pasta Sauce, tomato based		47.0	2.0	6.9	1.5	N
Pasta Sauce						
with bacon	Napolina	62.0	2.6	9.4	1.5	n/a
with mushrooms	Napolina	48.0	1.3	7.2	1.7	n/a
with peppers	Napolina	60.0	1.8	9.5	1.6	n/a
with tomato & herbs	Napolina	62.0	2.6	9.4	1.5	n/a
Pasta Shells with Vegetables & Prawns	Heinz Weight Watchers	76.0	4.7	10.1	1.9	0.7
Pastiles: *see flavours*						
Pastilles		253	5.2	61.9	nil	nil
Pastries: *see flavours*						
Pastry						
flaky, cooked		560	5.6	45.9	40.6	1.4
shortcrust, cooked		521	6.6	54.2	32.3	2.2
wholemeal, cooked		499	8.9	44.6	32.9	6.3
Pastry Mix	Whitworths	484	7.1	58.5	26.2	2.6
Pate: *see flavours*						

Patent Cornflour	Brown & Polson	330	0.4	87.4	0.1	n/a
Pavlova: *see flavours*						
Paw-paw, raw		36.0	0.5	8.8	0.1	2.2
canned in juice		65.0	0.2	17.0	Tr	0.7
Pea & Ham Soup	Baxters	75.0	3.1	9.7	2.9	1.5
	Heinz Whole Soups	54.0	3.5	8.9	0.5	1.6
Peach & Goldenberry Tropical Yogurt	St Ivel Shape	42.0	4.7	6.1	0.1	n/a
Peach & Papaya Soya Dessert	Granose	95.0	1.3	14.7	3.8	n/a
Peach & Passionfruit Fromage Frais Split	Ski Gold	134	5.5	17.4	5.2	n/a
Peach & Passionfruit Slice	Boots Shapers	198	5.2	27.0	8.5	1.2
Peach & Passionfruit Yogurt extrafruit	Ski	88.0	4.9	16.6	0.7	n/a
fruit on bottom, bio	Ski	116	5.4	16.0	2.8	n/a
Peach & Praline Real Fruit Le Yogurt, stirred, low fat	Chamboury	95.0	5.1	16.7	0.9	0.1

All amounts given per 100g/100ml unless otherwise stated

Product	Brand	Calories kcal	Protein (g)	Carbohydrate (g)	Fat (g)	Dietary Fibre (g)
Peach & Raspberries Yogurt, Greek Style	St Ivel Prize	133	3.7	15.0	6.6	n/a
Peach & Raspberry Layer Pies, each	Mr Kipling	203	2.1	33.7	2.1	n/a
Peach Chutney	Sharwood	164	0.4	41.3	0.2	0.8
Peach Fromage Frais	Ski	138	6.7	14.0	6.5	n/a
Peach Fruit Swirl	Ski	111	4.6	16.2	3.5	n/a
Peach Halves						
in natural juice	Libby	51.0	0.4	12.4	Tr	0.3
in syrup	Libby	82.0	0.5	20.0	Tr	0.3
Peach Melba Ice Cream	Lyons Maid	94.0	1.7	13.2	3.8	n/a
Peach Melba Soya Yogurt	Granose	73.0	3.0	11.4	1.8	n/a
Peach Melba Yogurt	Ski	86.0	4.7	16.2	0.7	nil
French style	St Ivel Shape	42.0	4.7	5.6	0.1	nil
long life	St Ivel Shape	40.0	4.8	5.3	0.1	nil
pasteurised, very low fat	St Ivel Prize	62.0	3.5	12.6	0.1	nil
	Dairy Crest	91.0	3.8	19.2	0.4	nil

Peach Slices						
in natural juice	Libby	52.0	0.4	12.4	0.1	0.3
in syrup	Libby	82.0	0.4	20.0	Tr	0.3
Peach Trifle	St Ivel	145	1.2	23.7	5.7	n/a
Peach Yogurt						
frozen	Ski	89.0	5.0	16.6	0.7	n/a
	Ski	129	3.7	27.2	1.4	n/a
low calorie	Diet Ski	35.0	3.9	4.8	0.2	n/a
Peaches						
raw		33.0	1.0	7.6	0.1	1.5
canned in natural juice		39.0	0.6	9.7	Tr	0.8
canned in syrup		55.0	0.5	14.0	Tr	0.9
Peaches & Cream Dairy Ice Cream	Boots Shapers	90.0	2.6	13.0	3.4	Tr
Peanut Butter, smooth		623	22.6	13.1	53.7	5.4
Peanut Butter/Crumble	Granose	586	28.1	8.6	49.0	n/a
Peanut Crunch Cake	Lyons	481	6.4	64.4	23.7	2.0
Peanut Crunchies, diabetic	Boots	502	11.0	52.0	32.0	2.2
Peanut Harvest Crunch Bar,						

All amounts given per 100g/100ml unless otherwise stated

Product	Brand	Calories kcal	Protein (g)	Carbo-hydrate (g)	Fat (g)	Dietary Fibre (g)
each	Quaker	86.0	1.9	9.9	4.6	0.6
Peanut M & Ms: see M & Ms						
Peanut Oil		899	Tr	nil	99.9	nil
Peanuts						
plain, kernel only		564	25.6	12.5	46.1	6.2
dry roasted		589	25.5	10.3	49.8	6.4
roasted & salted		602	24.5	7.1	53.0	6.0
Pear & Apple Juice	Copella	39.0	n/a	10.1	nil	nil
Pear & Raspberry Extrafruit Yogurt	Ski	87.0	5.6	15.6	0.7	n/a
Pear Drops, each	Trebor Bassett	15.0	n/a	4.0	n/a	n/a
Pear Halves						
in natural juice	Libby	54.0	0.1	13.3	Tr	0.5
in syrup	Libby	77.0	0.1	19.2	Tr	0.6
Pearl Barley, boiled	Whitworths	120	2.7	27.6	0.6	2.2
Pears						
raw, average		40.0	0.3	10.0	0.1	2.2

canned in natural juice		33.0	0.3	8.5	Tr	1.4
canned in syrup		50.0	0.2	13.2	Tr	1.1
Peas (see also products & varieties)						
boiled		79.0	6.7	10.0	1.6	4.5
dried, boiled		109	6.9	19.9	0.8	5.5
frozen, boiled		69.0	6.0	9.7	0.9	5.1
canned		80.0	5.3	13.5	0.9	5.1
Peas & Baby Carrots, 1oz/28g	Birds Eye	10.0	1.0	1.5	Tr	n/a
Pecan Nuts		689	9.2	5.8	70.1	4.7
Peking Barbecue Cook-In-Sauce	Homepride	103	0.3	22.5	n/a	n/a
Peking Barbecue Spare Ribs	Knorr	85.0	0.8	18.9	1.2	0.5
Penguin Biscuits	McVitie's	448	5.3	70.0	16.5	1.1
Pepper Pate						
per tub	Tartex	215	6.0	9.0	17.0	0.4
	Vessen	97.0	2.7	4.1	7.8	0.2
Pepper Relish	Branston	125	0.7	31.7	0.3	1.0
Peppercorn Pate, reduced calorie	Boots Shapers	184	17.0	4.5	11.0	n/a

All amounts given per 100g/100ml unless otherwise stated

Product	Brand	Calories kcal	Protein (g)	Carbo-hydrate (g)	Fat (g)	Dietary Fibre (g)
Peppered Grillsteak	Ross	328	11.8	4.6	29.2	0.2
Peppermint Chewing Gum (Wrigley): see Chewing Gum						
Peppermint Cordial, diluted	Britvic	18.0	n/a	4.9	n/a	n/a
Peppermint Cream, per bar	Cadbury	215	1.5	36.9	7.7	n/a
Peppermint Flavour Milk Chocolate, diabetic	Boots	471	9.9	51.0	32.0	2.6
Peppermints		392	0.5	102.2	0.7	nil
Pepperoni Deep Pan Pizza	McCain Pizza Perfection	218	10.5	27.0	8.3	n/a
Pepperoni French Bread Pizza	Heinz Weight Watchers	152	10.5	14.7	5.7	2.3
Pepperoni, Ham & Spicy Beef Micro Pizza	McCain Pizza Perfection	206	12.7	29.7	4.8	n/a
Pepperoni Pizza Slice	McCain Pizza Pantry	172	8.1	28.3	3.7	n/a
Peppers green, raw		15.0	0.8	2.6	0.3	1.6

green, boiled		18.0	1.0	2.6	0.5	1.8
red, raw		32.0	1.0	6.4	0.4	1.6
red, boiled		34.0	1.1	7.0	0.4	1.7
yellow, raw		26.0	1.2	5.3	0.2	1.7
Perkins	Tunnock's	429	7.4	77.4	12.0	n/a
Perry	Bulmer	43.0	n/a	n/a	n/a	n/a
Petits Pois, frozen, boiled		49.0	5.0	5.5	0.9	4.5
canned		45.0	5.2	4.9	0.6	4.3
Pheasant, roast, meat only		213	32.2	nil	9.3	nil
Philadelphia Full Fat Soft Cheese, all flavours	Kraft	313	8.0	3.0	30.0	n/a
Philadelphia Light Medium Fat Soft Cheese	Kraft	198	12.0	4.0	15.0	n/a
with pineapple	Kraft	185	7.6	12.6	11.4	n/a
with salmon	Kraft	190	10.0	4.0	15.0	n/a
Piccalilli	Heinz Ploughman's	90.0	1.0	21.5	Tr	1.0
Pickle, sweet		134	0.6	34.4	0.3	1.2

All amounts given per 100g/100ml unless otherwise stated

Product	Brand	Calories kcal	Protein (g)	Carbo-hydrate (g)	Fat (g)	Dietary Fibre (g)
	Heinz					
	Ploughman's	116	0.8	28.2	Tr	1.3
	Branston	150	0.7	34.5	0.2	1.7
Pickled Beetroot: see Beetroot						
Pickled Onion Crisps, per pack	Golden Wonder	150	2.0	12.2	10.6	n/a
Pickled Onions: see Onions						
Pickled Gherkin: see Gherkin						
Picnic, per bar	Cadbury	235	5.2	25.4	13.5	n/a
Pie Filling Mixes: see flavours						
Pigeon, roast, meat only		230	27.8	nil	13.2	nil
Pikelets	Mothers Pride	199	5.7	34.3	5.6	1.2
Pilau Rice	Batchelors	362	8.9	77.2	4.0	n/a
	Sharwood	365	8.6	76.8	1.2	1.8
frozen	Uncle Ben's	147	3.0	30.3	2.4	n/a
Pilchards, canned in tomato sauce		126	18.8	0.7	5.4	Tr

Pinacolada Fromage Frais	St Ivel Shape	54.0	6.8	6.5	0.2	n/a
Pine Nuts		688	14.0	4.0	68.6	1.9
Pineapple						
raw		41.0	0.4	10.1	0.2	1.2
canned in natural juice		47.0	0.3	12.2	Tr	0.5
canned in syrup		64.0	0.5	16.5	Tr	0.7
Pineapple & Clementine Fromage Frais	Ski	139	6.7	14.2	6.5	n/a
Pineapple & Clementine Fruit Swirl	Ski	112	4.6	16.5	3.5	n/a
Pineapple & Coconut Yogurt	Boots Shapers	42.0	4.3	6.5	0.1	Tr
Pineapple & Cream Mivvi, each	Lyons Maid	87.0	1.2	13.9	2.9	n/a
Pineapple & Orange Le Yogurt Actif, stirred	Chambourcy	104	4.3	14.7	3.1	0.2
Pineapple 'C'	Libby	44.0	0.1	10.9	Tr	Tr
Pineapple Chunks, each	Trebor Bassett	17.0	n/a	4.5	n/a	n/a
Pineapple Chunks in Juice	Del Monte	63.0	0.4	16.0	0.2	n/a

All amounts given per 100g/100ml unless otherwise stated

Product	Brand	Calories kcal	Protein (g)	Carbo-hydrate (g)	Fat (g)	Dietary Fibre (g)
Pineapple Cottage Cheese	Eden Vale Fruity	97.0	11.0	7.3	2.9	n/a
diet	St Ivel Shape	71.0	10.8	6.4	0.4	n/a
	Eden Vale Bodyline	82.0	11.1	6.1	1.6	n/a
Pineapple Crusha	Burgess	118	nil	28.7	nil	nil
Pineapple Fromage Frais	Diet Ski	71.0	8.1	6.7	1.5	n/a
Pineapple Fruit Juice	Del Monte	46.0	0.3	11.9	Tr	n/a
Pineapple Juice, unsweetened		41.0	0.3	10.5	0.1	Tr
Pineapple Melbas	Lyons	386	2.4	68.9	13.1	0.9
Pineapple Rings in Syrup	Libby	80.0	0.4	19.6	Tr	0.4
Pineapple Yogurt	Ski	89.0	5.0	16.7	0.7	n/a
Pinto Beans, dried, boiled refried		137	8.9	23.9	0.7	N
		107	6.2	15.3	1.1	N
Pistachio Nuts, weighed with shells		331	9.9	4.6	30.5	3.3
Pitta Bread, white wholemeal	Allinson	265	9.2	57.9	1.2	2.2
		227	1.21	41.5	1.8	7.1

Pizza: *see flavours*

Pizza Base Mix, as sold	Homepride Perfect	276	10.0	52.0	2.5	nil
Pizza Bases	Napolina	282	8.5	55.8	4.1	n/a
Pizza Classica, each mozzarella & vegetables	Birds Eye Gino Ginelli	620	22.0	67.0	31.0	n/a
mozzarella, ham & pineapple	Birds Eye Gino Ginelli	750	30.0	57.0	40.0	n/a
Pizza Quattro, each ham, mushroom & sweetcorn	Birds Eye Gino Ginelli	315	16.0	43.0	10.0	n/a
pepperoni	Birds Eye Gino Ginelli	400	19.0	42.0	18.0	n/a
Pizza Style Cheese	St Ivel	390	24.6	0.4	32.6	n/a
Pizza Toppings tomato, cheese, onion & herbs	Napolina	78.0	2.1	10.1	3.4	n/a
tomato, herbs & spices	Napolina	64.0	1.3	11.3	1.8	n/a

All amounts given per 100g/100ml unless otherwise stated

Product	Brand	Calories kcal	Protein (g)	Carbo- hydrate (g)	Fat (g)	Dietary Fibre (g)
PK Chewing Gum (Wrigley): see flavours						
Plaice, steamed		93.0	18.9	nil	1.9	nil
in batter, fried in oil		279	15.8	14.4	18.0	N
in crumbs, fried, fillets		228	18.0	8.6	13.7	N
Plaice Fillets	Ross Fish Shop	91.0	17.9	nil	2.2	n/a
boneless	Ross Chip Shop	191	12.2	16.7	8.7	0.7
breaded	Ross Fish Shop	127	12.9	16.0	1.4	0.7
Plaice Florentine	Heinz Weight Watchers	94.0	8.7	6.9	3.5	2.0
Plain Chocolate		525	4.7	64.8	29.2	N
diabetic	Boots	461	6.1	57.0	31.0	2.0
Plain Chocolate Coated Mixed Nut Cereal Bar	Boots Shapers	490	8.5	52.0	29.0	4.6
Plain Club Biscuits	Jacob's	499	4.4	63.0	27.2	0.8
Plain Devon Scones	Mothers Pride	350	7.4	49.2	13.1	1.9
Plain Superfine Chocolate	Rowntree Mackintosh	504	3.6	58.8	29.9	n/a

Plain Yogurt, pasteurised, very low fat	Dairy Crest	53.0	4.7	7.9	0.5	nil
PLJ Lemon Juice, undiluted	SmithKline Beecham	25.0	0.3	2.3	n/a	n/a
Ploughman's Pickles, Sauces, etc (Heinz); *see flavours*						
Plum & Apple Thick & Creamy Yogurt	Boots	108	4.3	17.0	3.0	n/a
Plum Custard Style Yogurt	Boots	138	4.2	19.0	5.5	n/a
Plums, average, raw		36.0	0.6	8.8	0.1	1.6
canned in syrup		59.0	0.3	15.5	Tr	0.8
Polar Mints, each	Trebor Bassett	19.0	n/a	5.0	n/a	n/a
Polka Dots milk chocolate	Lyons Tetley	487	9.0	61.0	24.7	1.9
plain chocolate	Lyons Tetley	503	3.9	63.6	27.6	2.7
Polo Fruits	Rowntree Mackintosh	368	nil	98.0	nil	n/a
Polo Mints	Rowntree Mackintosh	378	1.1	97.2	1.1	n/a

All amounts given per 100g/100ml unless otherwise stated

Product	Brand	Calories kcal	Protein (g)	Carbohydrate (g)	Fat (g)	Dietary Fibre (g)
Polony		281	9.4	14.2	21.1	N
Pomagne						
medium dry	Bulmer	46.0	n/a	n/a	n/a	n/a
medium sweet	Bulmer	56.0	n/a	n/a	n/a	n/a
rosé	Bulmer	40.0	n/a	n/a	n/a	n/a
Pontefract Cakes	Trebor Bassett	290	2.2	70.7	0.2	0.6
Popcorn, candied		480	2.1	77.6	20.0	N
plain		592	6.2	48.6	42.8	N
Poppadums	Sharwood	295	17.7	58.5	0.5	7.9
fried in veg. oil		369	17.5	39.1	16.9	N
Popular Pies (Lyons): see flavours						
Pork, belly rashers						
lean & fat, grilled		398	21.1	nil	34.8	nil
Pork, chops						
loin, lean only, grilled		226	32.3	nil	10.7	nil
Pork, leg						
lean & fat, roast		286	26.9	nil	19.8	nil

		kcal	g	g	g	g
lean only, roast		185	30.7	nil	6.9	nil
Pork, trotters & tails salted, boiled		280	19.8	nil	22.3	nil
Pork & Apple Casserole Cook In The Pot Dry Mix, as sold	Crosse & Blackwell	408	3.5	58.6	20.0	0.4
Pork Casserole Mix, as sold	Colman's	309	6.6	n/a	1.4	n/a
Pork Cubes	Knorr	348	9.3	27.3	23.1	0.5
Pork Pie, individual		376	9.8	24.9	27.0	0.9
Pork Roll, stuffed, canned	Tyne Brand	153	10.7	9.6	8.3	n/a
Pork Sausages: see Sausages						
Pork Spare Ribs with Peking Sauce	Heinz	464	11.3	7.3	4.0	0.1
Porridge, made with water	Whitworths	49.0	1.5	9.0	1.0	0.8
made with whole milk		116	4.8	13.7	5.1	0.8
Porridge Oats, cooked	Whitworths	44.0	1.4	8.2	0.9	0.8
uncooked	Whitworths	401	12.4	72.8	8.7	7.0

All amounts given per 100g/100ml unless otherwise stated

Product	Brand	Calories kcal	Protein (g)	Carbohydrate (g)	Fat (g)	Dietary Fibre (g)
Port		157	0.1	12.0	nil	nil
Postman Pat Chews, each	Trebor Bassett	35.0	Tr	7.7	0.24	n/a
Potato & Chive Salad	Eden Vale	162	1.0	17.2	10.3	n/a
Potato & Frankfurter Salad	Boots	219	3.3	14.0	17.0	0.5
	St Ivel Shape	140	2.5	14.1	8.6	n/a
Potato & Garlic Soup with Mushrooms	Baxters	41.0	1.2	8.3	0.6	0.5
Potato & Ham Gratin	Findus Dinner Supreme	118	6.4	6.5	7.6	1.9
Potato & Leek Soup	Baxters	36.0	0.6	7.1	0.7	0.8
	Heinz Farmhouse	36.0	0.8	7.0	0.5	0.6
Potato & Pea Curry	Sharwood	106	2.9	9.9	6.0	3.0
Potato Cakes	Mothers Pride	178	3.9	35.9	1.6	3.2
	Sunblest	255	4.6	32.7	11.7	1.9
Potato Crisps (see also flavours)		546	5.6	49.3	37.6	4.9
low fat		483	6.6	63.0	21.5	6.3

Potato Croquettes, fried in oil						
each	Ross	214	3.7	21.6	13.1	1.3
	Birds Eye	107	2.7	24.3	0.5	1.5
Fry Fresh		30.0	0.5	5.0	1.0	n/a
	McCain	96.0	2.3	23.0	n/a	n/a
Potato Fritters, crispy, 1oz/28g	Birds Eye	60.0	1.0	7.5	3.0	n/a
Potato Hoops		523	3.9	58.5	32.0	2.6
Potato Ketchips, 1oz/28g	Birds Eye	60.0	1.0	7.5	3.0	n/a
Potato Pancakes	Ross	183	3.9	20.6	10.1	1.6
Potato Powder: see Instant Potato Powder						
Potato Salad	Heinz	172	1.8	17.0	10.8	1.2
	St Ivel Shape	125	1.3	13.5	7.7	n/a
Potato Scones	Allinson	208	3.5	26.8	5.2	5.4
	Mothers Pride	178	3.9	35.9	1.6	3.2
Potato Waffles, frozen, cooked						
each	Ross	200	3.2	30.3	8.2	2.3
	Birds Eye	209	2.4	23.5	12.3	1.2
with cheese, each	Birds Eye	115	1.0	15.0	6.0	n/a
	Birds Eye	105	1.5	13.0	5.5	n/a
Potatoes, new boiled		75.0	1.5	17.8	0.3	1.1

All amounts given per 100g/100ml unless otherwise stated

Product	Brand	Calories kcal	Protein (g)	Carbo-hydrate (g)	Fat (g)	Dietary Fibre (g)
boiled in skins		66.0	1.4	15.4	0.3	1.5
canned		63.0	1.5	15.1	0.1	0.8
Potatoes, old						
baked, flesh & skin		136	3.9	31.7	0.2	2.7
baked, flesh only		77.0	2.2	18.0	0.1	1.4
boiled		72.0	1.8	17.0	0.1	1.2
mashed with margarine & milk		104	1.8	15.5	4.3	1.1
roast in oil/lard		149	2.9	25.9	4.5	1.8
Potted Shrimps	Young's	361	16.4	nil	32.8	n/a
Pour Over Sauces (Knorr): *see flavours*						
Pouring Syrup (Lyle's): *see flavours*						
Praline Ice Cream	Wall's Carte D'Or	145	2.5	15.0	9.0	n/a
Praline Viennetta	Wall's	140	2.1	13.8	8.8	n/a
Prawn Cocktail	Lyons	400	5.7	1.8	39.7	n/a
luxury	Lyons	407	6.0	2.6	43.9	n/a
Prawn Cocktail Crisps, per bag	Golden Wonder	151	2.0	12.1	10.5	n/a

278

Prawn Cocktail Sauce	Burgess	362	2.2	17.3	30.8	0.4
Prawn Crackers	Sharwood	296	1.0	69.4	0.5	1.7
Prawn Crumble Fast Cook	Ross Recipe Meal	163	8.2	14.2	8.4	0.6
Prawn Curry	Findus Dinner Supreme	110	4.3	18.0	2.3	0.8
Prawn Curry with Rice, per pack	Birds Eye Menu Master	370	13.0	68.0	7.0	n/a
	Findus Lean Cuisine	276	15.3	36.9	7.5	3.3
Prawn Nuggets, Golden	Young's	175	11.5	11.1	9.6	0.5
Prawn Provencale	Heinz Weight Watchers	81.0	5.2	12.4	1.2	0.8
Prawn Risotto Fast Cook	Ross Recipe Meal	103	5.1	17.3	1.8	0.7
Prawn Salad	Eden Vale	145	4.9	7.4	10.9	n/a
	St Ivel Shape	124	3.7	4.4	10.3	n/a
Prawnmaise (Lyons): *see flavours*						
Prawns, boiled		107	22.6	nil	1.8	nil

All amounts given per 100g/100ml unless otherwise stated

Product	Brand	Calories kcal	Protein (g)	Carbohydrate (g)	Fat (g)	Dietary Fibre (g)
cooked & peeled	Lyons	53.0	12.0	nil	0.6	n/a
Preserving Sugar	Tate & Lyle	394	nil	99.9	nil	nil
Prime Fish Steaks, per pack in butter sauce	Birds Eye	145	15.0	9.0	5.5	n/a
in cheese & tomato sauce	Captain's Table	190	18.0	7.0	10.0	n/a
in mushroom, cream & wine sauce	Birds Eye	215	18.0	9.0	12.0	n/a
in parsley sauce	Captain's Table	135	15.0	9.5	4.5	n/a
in traditional batter	Birds Eye / Captain's Table	215	13.0	12.0	13.0	n/a
Primula Cheese Spread						
original	Kavli	255	16.0	1.0	21.0	n/a
with celery	Kavli	255	16.0	1.0	21.0	n/a
with chives	Kavli	255	15.0	1.5	21.0	n/a
with crab	Kavli	255	16.0	1.0	21.0	n/a
with ham	Kavli	253	15.0	1.0	21.0	n/a
with onion	Kavli	251	14.0	1.5	21.0	n/a

with shrimp	Kavli	253	15.0	1.0	21.0	n/a
Primula Light Dairy Spread						
with cheese	Kavli	164	16.0	5.0	9.0	n/a
with cheese & ham	Kavli	164	16.0	5.0	9.0	n/a
with cheese, garlic & herbs	Kavli	175	20.0	4.0	9.0	n/a
Primula Low Fat Dairy Spread						
with cheese	Kavli	164	16.0	5.0	9.0	n/a
with cheese, garlic & herbs	Kavli	164	16.0	5.0	9.0	n/a
with cheese & mixed seafood	Kavli	175	20.0	4.0	9.0	n/a
Prizebake White Bread	Mothers Pride	235	8.6	41.3	3.2	2.9
Prizeburgers, each	Birds Eye Steakhouse	210	20.0	3.0	13.0	n/a
Prizegrill Platter, per pack	Birds Eye MenuMaster	520	28.0	41.0	28.0	n/a
Prizegrills, each	Birds Eye Steakhouse	195	19.0	1.0	13.0	n/a

All amounts given per 100g/100ml unless otherwise stated

Product	Brand	Calories kcal	Protein (g)	Carbohydrate (g)	Fat (g)	Dietary Fibre (g)
Processed Cheese, plain						
cheddar slices	Kraft	330	20.8	0.9	27.0	nil
singles slices	Kraft	326	22.0	1.0	26.0	n/a
slices, reduced fat	Heinz Weight Watchers	300	20.0	1.0	24.0	n/a
		197	26.5	0.2	10.0	nil
Processed Peas, canned		99.0	6.9	17.5	0.7	4.8
Profiteroles	McVitie's	470	7.6	21.6	39.3	0.9
Provencale Cook-In-Sauce	Homepride	47.0	1.2	9.4	n/a	n/a
Provencale Rice	Batchelors	365	7.9	77.9	4.6	n/a
Prune Fruit Snack Bar, each	Granose	77.5	1.2	16.5	1.0	2.0
Prunes						
canned in juice		79.0	0.7	19.7	0.2	2.4
canned in syrup		90.0	0.6	23.0	0.2	2.8
ready to eat		141	2.5	34.0	0.4	5.7
Puffed Wheat		321	14.2	67.3	1.3	5.6
Pumpkin, raw		13.0	0.7	2.2	0.2	1.0
boiled		13.0	0.6	2.1	0.3	1.1

Quakeawake Summer Fruit	Quaker	420	9.3	73.3	11.5	5.7
Quaker Oat Bran	Quaker	339	16.8	53.0	7.6	14.5
Quaker Oat Bran Crispies	Quaker	362	13.9	67.5	5.3	9.0
Quaker Oat Bran Muesli	Quaker	353	11.2	64.8	6.9	8.7
Quaker Oats	Quaker	375	10.0	70.2	7.4	7.0
with oat bran	Quaker	356	11.9	63.7	7.6	9.2
Quality Street, assortment 100g bag	Rowntree	444	3.6	72.2	17.6	n/a
	Mackintosh	458	4.0	69.5	20.1	n/a
Quarter Pounder each	Birds Eye Steakhouse	235	17.0	3.5	17.0	n/a
each	McDonald's	400	26.3	39.0	16.4	3.3

All amounts given per 100g/100ml unless otherwise stated

283

Product	Brand	Calories kcal	Protein (g)	Carbohydrate (g)	Fat (g)	Dietary Fibre (g)
chilli beef, each	Birds Eye Steakhouse	195	15.0	3.5	12.0	n/a
lean beef	Findus	180	15.2	2.7	12.0	0.2
with cheese, each	McDonald's	492	34.0	40.1	22.9	3.8
Queen of Puddings	McVitie's	203	4.8	26.5	8.7	0.2
Quenchers	Trebor Bassett	332	3.6	80.0	nil	nil
Quiche (see also flavours)						
cheese & egg		314	12.5	17.3	22.2	0.6
cheese & egg, wholemeal		308	13.2	14.5	22.4	1.9
Quick Batter Mix	Whitworths	338	9.3	77.2	1.2	3.7
Quick Jel Dessert Mix, all flavours, as sold	Green's	133	Tr	35.0	Tr	n/a
Quorn, myco-protein		86.0	11.8	2.0	3.5	4.8
Quosh Fruit Drinks: see flavours						

R

Rabbit, stewed, meat only		179	27.3	nil	7.7	nil
Raddiccio, raw		14.0	1.4	1.7	0.2	1.8
Radish, red, raw		12.0	0.7	1.9	0.2	0.9
white/mooli, raw		15.0	0.8	2.9	0.1	N
Ragu Pasta Sauces (Brooke Bond): *see flavours*						
Rainbow Trout	Young's	147	16.9	n/a	8.8	n/a
Raisin & Biscuit Chocolate	Rowntree Mackintosh	470	7.3	60.0	24.0	n/a
Raisin & Biscuit Yorkie	Rowntree Mackintosh	460	6.7	59.5	23.3	n/a
Raisin & Lemon Pancakes	Sunblest	274	5.9	49.0	6.0	2.1

All amounts given per 100g/100ml unless otherwise stated

Product	Brand	Calories kcal	Protein (g)	Carbohydrate (g)	Fat (g)	Dietary Fibre (g)
Raisin Bran Buns	Vitbe	315	4.9	46.3	12.2	5.3
Raisin Fruit Snack Bar, each	Granose	85.0	1.0	17.7	1.0	2.0
Raisin Fudge, each	Trebor Bassett	40.0	n/a	6.5	1.6	n/a
Raisin Harvest Crunch Bar, each	Quaker	78.0	1.3	11.4	3.3	0.7
Raisin Splitz	Kellogg's	340	9.0	70.0	2.0	8.0
Raisins		272	2.1	69.3	0.4	2.0
seedless	Whitworths	300	3.2	79.1	0.5	1.3
stoned	Whitworths	275	1.7	68.1	1.4	4.4
Raisins & Peanuts		435	15.3	37.5	26.0	4.4
Rambutans & Pineapple in Syrup	Libby	74.0	n/a	n/a	Tr	n/a
Rapeseed Oil		899	Tr	nil	99.9	nil
Raspberries, raw		7.0	0.9	0.8	0.1	2.5
stewed with sugar		48.0	0.9	11.5	0.1	1.2
stewed without sugar		7.0	0.9	0.7	0.1	1.3
canned in syrup		31.0	0.5	7.6	Tr	0.8

Raspberry & Apple Pies, each	Mr Kipling	179	2.0	28.9	7.0	n/a
Raspberry & Cream Mivvi, each	Lyons Maid	87.0	1.2	13.9	2.9	n/a
Raspberry & Lemon Le Yogurt Actif, stirred	Chambourcy	105	4.3	14.7	3.2	0.4
Raspberry & Passionfruit Thick & Creamy Yogurt	Boots	107	5.0	16.0	3.0	n/a
Raspberry & Redcurrant Creme Brulee	McVitie's	251	1.3	23.5	17.0	0.2
Raspberry & Vanilla Swiss Roll	Lyons	322	4.2	61.5	8.3	1.4
Raspberry Blancmange	Brown & Polson	330	0.4	87.4	0.1	n/a
Raspberry Cheesecake individual	Eden Vale Young's	261 235	2.8 6.0	38.8 23.7	11.6 13.1	n/a 0.4
Raspberry Crusha	Burgess	113	0.1	27.3	nil	nil
Raspberry Fresta	Wall's	80.0	2.0	14.0	2.5	n/a
Raspberry Fromage Frais	St Ivel Shape	49.0	6.8	5.2	0.2	n/a
Raspberry Fruit Snack						

All amounts given per 100g/100ml unless otherwise stated

Product	Brand	Calories kcal	Protein (g)	Carbo-hydrate (g)	Fat (g)	Dietary Fibre (g)
Bar, each	Granose	87.0	0.7	17.0	1.7	1.7
Raspberry Jam						
diabetic	Applefords	100	0.2	19.5	Tr	n/a
	Boots	156	0.5	62.0	nil	2.3
	Dietade	249	0.2	66.1	n/a	n/a
reduced sugar	Heinz Weight Watchers	125	0.4	33.0	Tr	3.7
Raspberry Jam Sponge Pudding	Heinz	297	2.6	49.4	9.9	0.8
Raspberry Jelly Crystals						
diabetic	Dietade	8.0	1.5	0.2	n/a	n/a
	Boots	340	65.0	20.0	Tr	nil
Raspberry Jelly, ready to eat	Rowntree	81.0	0.1	20.2	Tr	0.8
Raspberry Juice	Hycal	243	nil	64.7	n/a	n/a
Raspberry Pavlova	McVitie's	336	2.3	34.2	21.1	Tr
Raspberry Preserve	Baxters	200	Tr	53.0	Tr	4.1
Raspberry Ripple Ice Cream	Wall's Gino Ginelli	95.0	1.5	15.0	3.5	n/a
reduced calorie	Heinz Weight					

	Watchers	71.0	1.5	8.6	2.5	0.1
Raspberry Ripple Soya Ice Cream	Granose	94.0	1.2	13.8	3.4	n/a
Raspberry Swiss Roll	Lyons	289	4.7	67.1	2.0	1.7
Raspberry Torte	McVitie's	271	3.5	24.5	17.8	0.4
Raspberry Trifle	Eden Vale	153	2.4	23.0	6.3	n/a
	St Ivel	144	1.3	23.2	5.7	n/a
Raspberry Yogurt						
custard style	Ski	87.0	5.0	16.3	0.7	nil
Fiendish Feet	Boots	125	4.1	17.0	5.0	n/a
long life	St Ivel	91.0	4.9	15.7	1.1	nil
low fat	St Ivel Prize	62.0	3.5	12.5	0.1	nil
	Diet Ski	35.0	3.9	4.8	0.2	nil
	Holland & Barrett	83.0	5.4	13.5	0.8	0.5
	St Ivel Shape	41.0	4.7	5.6	0.1	nil
	Dairy Crest	87.0	3.8	18.1	0.4	nil
pasteurised, very low fat						
Ratatouille, canned	Buitoni	45.0	1.3	5.3	1.9	0.9
Ratatouille Mix	Ross	72.0	2.9	13.6	0.9	0.6
Ravioli, canned	Granose	80.5	3.1	15.9	0.4	1.1

All amounts given per 100g/100ml unless otherwise stated

Product	Brand	Calories kcal	Protein (g)	Carbo-hydrate (g)	Fat (g)	Dietary Fibre (g)
in beef & tomato sauce	Heinz	79.0	3.5	13.3	1.3	0.5
in tomato sauce	Heinz	79.0	3.0	14.4	1.0	0.7
Ravioli Bianche	Dolmio	200	9.6	29.7	4.7	n/a
Raw Cane Demerara Sugar	Tate & Lyle	390	Tr	99.2	nil	Tr
Ready Brek	Weetabix	364	12.2	61.1	7.9	7.5
with chocolate	Weetabix	363	11.9	62.0	7.5	7.3
Ready Meals (Ross); see flavours						
Ready Salted Crisps, per pack	Golden Wonder	155	1.9	12.0	11.0	n/a
Ready-To-Roll Icing	Tate & Lyle	409	nil	89.0	6.4	nil
Real Chocolate Fancies, each	Mr Kipling	98.0	1.5	12.5	5.2	n/a
Real Chocolate Mousse	Chambourcy	189	4.8	25.8	7.4	0.3
Real Fruit Gums	Trebor Bassett	315	3.5	77.0	nil	nil
Real Fruit Jellies, each	Trebor Bassett	31.0	n/a	6.8	n/a	n/a
Real Fruit Pastilles	Trebor Bassett	331	3.2	81.3	nil	nil
Real Juice, Squash, Yogurt; etc: see also flavours						

Real Mayonnaise	Burgess Hellmanns	743 719	1.5 1.1	2.5 1.5	80.5 78.8	nil nil
Real White Chocolate Mousse	Chambourcy	193	5.7	23.1	8.6	nil
Recipe Meals (Knorr): *see flavours*						
Recipe Sauces (Knorr): *see flavours*						
Red Butterfly Rice Pudding	Fussell's	91.0	3.2	16.0	1.6	0.2
Red Cherry Cheesecake Mix made up, per serving	Homepride Classic	251	3.5	47.0	12.0	n/a
Red Cherry Crepes Mix made up, per serving	Homepride Classic	180	4.5	25.0	7.0	n/a
Red Kidney Beans, boiled canned		103 100	8.4 6.9	17.4 17.8	0.5 0.6	9.0 8.5
Red Leicester Cheese Spread, low fat	St Ivel Shape	153	12.0	6.3	9.0	n/a
Red Leicester Cheese Wedge	St Ivel Shape	262	29.1	0.1	16.1	n/a
Red Lentils: *see Lentils*						
Red Pepper Chutney	Baxters	120	0.7	30.1	0.3	0.6

All amounts given per 100g/100ml unless otherwise stated

Product	Brand	Calories kcal	Protein (g)	Carbo-hydrate (g)	Fat (g)	Dietary Fibre (g)
Red Peppers: see Peppers						
Red Wine		68.0	0.2	0.3	nil	nil
Red Wine & Herbs Ragu	Brooke Bond	84.0	1.9	12.1	2.8	n/a
Red Wine Casserole Sauce	Knorr	80.0	1.4	7.9	5.0	n/a
Red Wine Cook-In-Sauce						
can	Homepride	38.0	0.5	7.7	n/a	n/a
jar	Homepride	44.0	0.6	8.4	n/a	n/a
Redcurrant Jelly	Burgess	129	0.6	30.9	nil	nil
Redcurrant Sauce	Colman's	255	0.5	n/a	Tr	n/a
Reduced Calorie Dressing	Crosse & Blackwell Waistline	140	0.8	11.0	9.9	0.3
	Heinz Weight Watchers	148	1.3	17.5	8.1	Tr
Reduced Fat Spreads: see flavours						
Refreshers, each	Trebor Bassett	6.0	n/a	1.4	0.1	n/a
Refried Beans	Old El Paso	94.0	n/a	n/a	n/a	n/a

Revels	Mars	478	7.5	65.4	22.5	n/a
Rhubarb, stewed with sugar		48.0	0.9	11.5	0.1	1.2
stewed without sugar		7.0	0.9	0.7	0.1	1.3
canned in syrup		31.0	0.5	7.6	Tr	0.8
Rhubarb & Ginger Preserve	Baxters	200	Tr	53.0	Tr	1.7
Rhubarb Crunchy Dessert Mix, per serving	Green's	252	2.0	45.0	8.0	n/a
Rhubarb Yogurt, custard style	Boots	135	4.1	18.0	5.0	n/a
low fat	St Ivel Shape	42.0	4.9	5.4	0.1	n/a
Ribena, undiluted		228	0.1	60.8	nil	nil
Ribena Juice Drinks (SmithKline Beecham): *see flavours*						
Rice, boiled brown		141	2.6	32.1	1.1	0.8
white		138	2.6	30.9	1.3	0.1
Rice Cakes	Applefords	356	8.0	73.6	3.2	n/a
Rice Choice (Crosse & Blackwell): *see flavours*						
Rice Krispies		369	6.1	89.7	0.9	0.7

All amounts given per 100g/100ml unless otherwise stated

Product	Brand	Calories kcal	Protein (g)	Carbo-hydrate (g)	Fat (g)	Dietary Fibre (g)
Rice Pudding, canned		89.0	3.4	14.0	2.5	0.2
Rice Pudding, creamed low fat, no added sugar	Heinz Weight Watchers	75.0	3.7	12.4	1.3	0.2
Rich Beef Casserole Recipe Sauce	Knorr	38.0	1.2	8.2	0.3	n/a
Rich Chocolate Slices, each	Mr Kipling	135	1.6	19.8	6.0	n/a
Rich Fruit Cake: see Fruit Cake						
Rich Jam Roly Poly	Mr Kipling	203	3.8	46.0	11.7	n/a
Rich Water Biscuits	Jacob's	411	10.0	69.0	12.5	3.4
Rich Tea Biscuits	McVitie's	470	6.7	74.2	15.7	2.3
	Peek Frean	443	6.1	71.9	13.7	2.1
Rich Tea Fingers	McVitie's	466	6.8	75.7	14.5	2.3
Ricicles		381	4.3	95.7	0.5	0.4
Ripple, Galaxy	Mars	518	9.0	56.6	30.0	n/a
Risotto, plain		224	3.0	34.4	9.3	0.4
Risotto Rice	Whitworths	324	7.0	77.8	0.6	0.4

Rissolnut	Granose	376	20.3	54.3	11.7	7.3
Ritz Crackers	Jacob's	495	7.3	69.0	23.6	n/a
Riviera Gourmet Sauce	Rakusen	54.0	n/a	n/a	2.9	n/a
Roast Beef & Gravy, per pack	Birds Eye MenuMaster	90.0	15.0	3.0	2.0	n/a
Roast Beef in Gravy	Findus Dinner Supreme	84.0	14.0	2.4	2.1	nil
Roast Beef Platter, each	Birds Eye MenuMaster	395	32.0	46.0	10.5	n/a
Roast Chicken Crisps, per pack	Golden Wonder	153	2.1	12.4	10.5	n/a
Roast Chicken Platter, each	Birds Eye MenuMaster	490	36.0	40.0	22.0	n/a
Roast Ham Thick & Crunchy Crisps, per pack	Golden Wonder	146	1.8	15.3	9.1	n/a
Roast Turkey & Gravy, per pack	Birds Eye MenuMaster	220	39.0	4.5	5.5	n/a
Roast Turkey Platter, each	Birds Eye					

All amounts given per 100g/100ml unless otherwise stated

Product	Brand	Calories kcal	Protein (g)	Carbo-hydrate (g)	Fat (g)	Dietary Fibre (g)
	MenuMaster	380	22.0	44.0	14.0	n/a
Roasted Almond Oatbran Bar	Jordans	410	9.0	45.9	22.0	6.3
Rock Cake Mix, made up, per serving	Homepride Perfect	103	2.5	15.5	3.5	n/a
Roe						
cod, hard, fried		202	20.9	3.0	11.9	0.1
herring, soft, fried		244	21.1	4.7	15.8	N
Rogan Classic Curry Sauce	Homepride	86.0	2.1	10.2	n/a	n/a
Rogan Josh Classic Curry Sauce	Homepride	73.0	1.9	10.2	n/a	n/a
Rogan Josh Medium Curry Sauce	Colman's	45.0	1.5	n/a	0.6	n/a
	Sharwood	90.0	2.8	7.3	5.6	2.6
mix, as sold	Sharwood	189	10.4	12.6	1.08	21.4
Rolls: see Bread Rolls						
Rolo	Rowntree Mackintosh	444	4.7	64.7	2.30	n/a

Romana Spirals	Heinz	66.0	2.3	13.1	0.8	0.5
Romano Pasta Choice Dry Mix, as sold	Crosse & Blackwell	351	12.0	66.3	4.2	1.0
Romano Salad Dressing	Napolina	550	1.8	4.7	53.5	n/a
Romany Biscuits	Huntley & Palmer	462	5.5	64.3	22.0	1.4
Rosé Wine		71.0	0.1	2.5	nil	nil
Roses	Cadbury	480	4.7	65.2	24.2	n/a
Rosehip Syrup, undiluted		232	Tr	61.9	nil	nil
Rough Oatcakes, each	Paterson's	56.2	n/a	n/a	2.3	n/a
Rowntree Jelly Crystals, unsweetened, as sold, all flavours	Rowntree	225	56.4	nil	nil	nil
Royal Game Soup	Baxters	32.0	1.6	5.0	0.8	0.3
Ruffle Bar, each	Cadbury	130	0.7	19.9	5.9	n/a
Rum: *see* Spirits						
Rum & Raisin Dairy Ice	Lyons Maid					

All amounts given per 100g/100ml unless otherwise stated

Product	Brand	Calories kcal	Protein (g)	Carbohydrate (g)	Fat (g)	Dietary Fibre (g)
Cream	Napoli	94.0	1.7	15.0	3.3	n/a
Rum & Raisin Ice Cream	Wall's Gino Ginelli Tub	110	2.0	17.0	4.0	n/a
Rum Instant Chocolate Drink	Boots Shapers	325	17.0	49.0	8.1	2.6
Rump Steak: *see Beef*						
Runner Beans, boiled		18.0	1.2	2.3	0.5	3.1
Russchian	Schweppes	23.3	n/a	6.2	n/a	n/a
Rye Bread: *see Bread*						
Rye Crispbread		321	9.4	70.6	2.1	11.7
Rye Flour, *whole*		335	8.2	75.9	20.	11.7
Ryvita, per slice						
original	Ryvita	25.0	0.7	5.6	0.2	1.3
brown	Ryvita	25.0	0.7	5.6	0.2	1.3
extra bran	Ryvita	25.0	0.8	5.3	0.2	1.5
sesame	Ryvita	30.0	1.0	5.2	0.7	1.4

S

Safflower Oil		899	Tr	nil	99.9	nil
Saffron Rice, frozen	Uncle Ben's	136	3.3	31.0	0.7	n/a
Sage & Onion Stuffing	Whitworths	231	5.2	20.4	14.8	1.7
		342	10.4	69.3	4.5	3.9
Sago, creamed	Ambrosia	82.0	2.9	13.2	1.8	n/a
Sago Pudding	Whitworths	131	4.1	20.4	4.2	nil
Saithe: see Coley						
Salad Cream	Crosse &	348	1.5	16.7	31.0	N
reduced calorie	Blackwell	194	1.0	9.4	17.2	N
	Heinz	370	1.6	15.5	33.0	0.5
		347	1.4	22.9	27.9	Tr

All amounts given per 100g/100ml unless otherwise stated

Product	Brand	Calories kcal	Protein (g)	Carbohydrate (g)	Fat (g)	Dietary Fibre (g)
economy	Burgess	283	1.2	7.5	27.0	nil
Salad Mayonnaise	Burgess	579	2.4	8.1	59.2	nil
Salami		491	19.3	1.9	45.2	0.1
Salmon *steamed, flesh only* *canned* *smoked*		197 155 142	20.1 203. 25.4	nil nil nil	13.0 8.2 4.5	nil nil nil
Salmon & Asparagus	Heinz Weight Watchers	84.0	5.6	10.1	2.4	0.5
Salmon & Cucumber Cottage Cheese	Eden Vale	110	12.0	2.5	5.9	n/a
Salmon & Prawn Fricasee	Heinz Weight Watchers	86.0	6.6	7.4	3.3	0.7
Salmon & Shrimp Paste	Shippams	192	n/a	n/a	n/a	n/a
Salmon Fish Cakes, each	Birds Eye	90.0	5.0	8.0	4.5	n/a
Salmon Mornay	Boots Shapers Heinz Weight	115	10.0	5.7	5.8	2.2

	Watchers	98.0	7.6	6.1	4.8	1.0
Salmon Paste	Shippams	145	n/a	n/a	n/a	n/a
Salmon Tagliatelle	Boots Shapers	128	9.5	12.0	5.0	1.1
St Clements Drinks (Barr): see flavours						
Salsa Lasagne Sauce	Napolina	84.0	3.5	7.6	4.6	n/a
Salsify, *raw*		27.0	1.3	10.2	0.3	3.2
boiled		23.0	1.1	8.6	0.4	3.5
Salt & Vinegar crisps, per pack	Golden Wonder	151	1.9	12.2	10.5	n/a
Salt & Vinegar Potato Fritters, 1oz/28g	Birds Eye	60.0	1.0	7.5	3.0	n/a
Salt & Vinegar Ringos	Golden Wonder	84.0	1.5	13.3	3.0	n/a
Salted Cashew Nuts: see Cashew Nuts						
Salted Peanuts: see Peanuts						
Samosas, meat		593	5.1	17.9	56.1	1.2
vegetable		472	3.1	22.3	41.8	1.8
Sandwich Baps	Mothers Pride	264	8.7	48.6	3.0	1.4
Sandwich Biscuits		513	5.0	69.2	25.9	N

All amounts given per 100g/100ml unless otherwise stated

Product	Brand	Calories kcal	Protein (g)	Carbo-hydrate (g)	Fat (g)	Dietary Fibre (g)
Sandwich Cakes: *see flavours*						
Sandwich Cake Mixes: *see flavours*						
Sandwich Snack	Cadbury	510	6.9	65.0	26.5	n/a
Sandwich Spread						
cucumber	Heinz	207	1.2	22.5	12.5	1.1
	Heinz	187	1.3	19.6	11.5	0.7
spicy	Heinz	212	1.3	23.1	12.7	1.1
Sandwichmaker (Shippams): *see flavours*						
Sardine & Tomato Spread	Shippams	143	n/a	n/a	n/a	n/a
Sardines						
canned in tomato sauce		177	17.8	0.5	11.6	Tr
canned in oil, drained		217	23.7	nil	13.6	nil
	Young's	196	17.6	nil	13.9	n/a
Satay Sauce	Burgess	289	4.6	38.5	12.5	1.3
Satsumas, *flesh only*		36.0	0.9	8.5	0.1	1.3
Sauce A L'Orange Mix, *dry as sold*	Crosse & Blackwell Bonne Cuisine	367	4.5	71.7	6.9	0.5

Sauce Tartare: see Tartare Sauce

Saucy Beans	HP	76.0	5.4	12.2	0.6	7.3
Sauerkraut		9.0	1.1	1.1	Tr	2.2
Sausage & Bacon Casserole Cook In The Pot Dry Mix, as sold	Crosse & Blackwell	374	14.7	59.1	8.8	2.0
Sausage & Baked Beans Savoury Pancake	Findus	175	5.7	24.6	6.0	2.6
Sausage & Tomato Casserole Cook In The Pot, as sold	Crosse & Blackwell	357	1.9	5.8	8.5	2.5
Sausage Casserole, canned	Campbell's	111	3.2	11.1	6.3	1.0
Sausage Casserole Cooking Mix, traditional farmhouse	Colman's Colman's	323 323	13.4 7.3	n/a n/a	1.6 0.9	n/a n/a
Sausage Feast	Findus Dinner Supreme	166	6.2	15.0	9.0	2.1
Sausage Pot Recipe Sauce						

All amounts given per 100g/100ml unless otherwise stated

Product	Brand	Calories kcal	Protein (g)	Carbohydrate (g)	Fat (g)	Dietary Fibre (g)
Mix, as sold	Knorr	310	6.6	58.9	6.9	7.0
Sausage Rolls						
flaky pastry		477	7.1	32.3	36.4	1.2
short pastry		459	8.0	37.5	31.9	1.4
cocktail	Kraft	320	6.6	24.7	22.3	n/a
	Ross	239	6.7	16.9	16.4	0.7
giant size	Kraft	320	6.6	24.7	22.3	n/a
jumbo cut to size	Ross	200	8.7	13.2	12.8	0.6
king size	Kraft	320	6.6	24.7	22.3	n/a
light 'n' tasty	Kraft	266	8.1	24.5	15.8	n/a
Sausages, beef						
fried		269	12.9	14.9	18.0	0.7
grilled		265	13.0	15.2	17.3	0.7
Sausages, pork						
fried		317	13.8	11.0	24.5	0.7
grilled		318	13.3	11.5	24.6	0.7
low fat, fried		211	14.9	9.1	13.0	1.4
low fat, grilled		229	16.2	10.8	1.38	1.5
Sausages & Mash,	Birds Eye					

per pack						
Sausalatas	Granose	137	11.0	7.1	4.1	1.4
Sausfry	Granose	476	17.8	28.8	33.4	11.1
Sauté Potatoes	Findus	130	2.1	19.9	4.7	2.1
Saveloy		262	9.9	10.1	20.5	N
Saviand	Granose	198	19.7	8.4	9.8	1.5
Savoury Haddock Crepe	Ross Recipe Meal	156	8.2	14.2	8.4	0.6
Savoury Haddock Pie	Ross Recipe Meal	114	6.4	10.8	5.2	0.5
Savoury Mince, canned	Tyne Brand	86.0	9.8	13.4	7.3	0.6
Savoury Mince Recipe Sauce Mix, as sold	Knorr	286	8.4	52.2	6.2	4.0
Savoury Onion Potatoes & Sauce	Batchelors	324	7.7	73.3	2.0	n/a
Savoury Pizza Toast Topper	Heinz	84.0	3.7	8.4	4.0	0.8
Savoury Pudding	Granose	207	8.0	15.9	12.8	1.4
Savoury Rice (Batchelors): *see flavours*						

All amounts given per 100g/100ml unless otherwise stated

Product	Brand	Calories kcal	Protein (g)	Carbohydrate (g)	Fat (g)	Dietary Fibre (g)
Savoury Rice, cooked		142	2.9	26.3	3.5	1.4
Savoury Rolls with Tofu	Granose	164	6.0	21.0	6.0	n/a
Savoury White Sauce Mix	Knorr	362	8.7	64.3	9.5	2.0
Scampi in Breadcrumbs, frozen, fried						
as eaten		316	12.2	28.9	17.6	N
Golden	Lyons	208	8.0	25.0	8.8	n/a
	Young's	231	9.2	14.2	15.5	0.6
Scone Mix, made up, per serving	Homepride Perfect	130	2.5	20.5	4.0	n/a
Scones, fruit		316	7.3	52.9	9.8	N
plain		362	7.2	53.8	14.6	1.9
wholemeal		326	8.7	43.1	14.4	5.2
Scotch Broth	Baxters	39.0	1.2	6.4	1.1	0.8
	Campbell's Bumper Harvest	36.0	1.3	6.5	0.6	0.6
	Heinz Farmhouse	36.0	1.8	6.0	0.7	0.9
condensed	Campbell's	80.0	2.1	11.2	3.0	1.2
Scotch Eggs		251	12.0	13.1	17.1	N

Scotch Mince	Baxters	96.0	7.6	5.4	5.0	0.6
Scotch Orange Marmalade	Baxters	200	Tr	53.0	Tr	Tr
Scotch Pancakes	Baxters	292	5.8	43.6	11.7	1.4
Scotch Vegetable Soup	Baxters	26.0	0.6	5.2	0.5	0.8
Scotch Whisky: see Whisky						
Scottish Game Soup	Campbell's	51.0	2.5	6.5	1.7	0.6
Scottish Haggis	Baxters	154	9.2	11.8	8.2	1.1
Scottish Lentil Soup	Crosse & Blackwell	44.0	2.6	6.2	1.0	1.0
Scottish Morning Rolls, each	Sunblest	122	4.5	22.6	1.5	0.8
Scottish Oatcakes, each	Paterson's	56.2	n/a	n/a	2.3	n/a
Scottish Salmon Slices	Young's	130	25.1	n/a	3.3	n/a
Scottish Salmon Steaks	Young's	130	25.1	nil	3.3	n/a
Scottish Vegetable Soup with Lentils	Heinz	45.0	3.1	7.0	0.5	1.7
Scotts Old Fashioned Oats	Quaker	375	10.0	70.2	7.4	7.0

All amounts given per 100g/100ml unless otherwise stated

Product	Brand	Calories kcal	Protein (g)	Carbo-hydrate (g)	Fat (g)	Dietary Fibre (g)
Scotts Piper Oatmeal	Quaker	375	10.0	70.2	7.4	7.0
Scotts Porage Oats	Quaker	375	10.0	70.2	7.4	7.0
Scrambled Eggs: see Eggs						
Scribbler, each	Wall's	25.0	Tr	6.0	Tr	n/a
Seafood & Chicken Paella, per pack	Birds Eye MenuMaster	335	29.0	45.0	5.5	n/a
Seafood Cocktail luxury	Lyons	81.0	13.0	4.0	1.5	n/a
	Lyons	81.0	14.9	1.3	2.3	n/a
Seafood Lasagne	Boots Shapers Heinz Weight Watchers	134	9.1	11.0	6.3	1.3
		74.0	6.1	8.2	1.9	0.4
Seafood Sauce	Colman's	387	0.8	n/a	35.0	n/a
Seafood Selection	Young's	226	8.6	27.5	9.6	1.1
Seafood Sticks	Young's	96.0	9.1	14.4	0.2	Tr
Secret	Rowntree Mackintosh	474	6.3	64.5	23.0	n/a

Seeded Burger Rolls, each	Sunblest	151	5.3	24.2	3.7	0.9
Semi-skimmed Milk: see Milk						
Semolina, creamed	Ambrosia	84.0	3.6.	13.2	1.9	n/a
Semolina Pudding	Whitworths	131	4.1	20.4	4.2	nil
Semolina Whisk & Serve, made up, per serving	Bird's	108	1.2	20.0	3.1	n/a
Sesame Chicken	Findus Lean Cuisine	117	8.0	15.8	2.4	1.6
Sesame Fruit Snack Bar, each	Granose	92.5	2.0	16.0	2.5	3.2
Sesame Oil		881	0.2	nil	99.7	nil
Shandy	Barr	27.0	n/a	n/a	n/a	n/a
	Corona	25.0	n/a	5.3	n/a	n/a
Shandy Bass	Barr	24.0	n/a	4.8	n/a	n/a
Shape Cheese Wedges (St Ivel): *see flavours*						
Shape Cottage Cheese (St Ivel): *see flavours*						
Shape Salads (St Ivel): *see flavours*						
Shape Milk Drink	St Ivel	45.0	3.8	5.5	10.5	n/a

All amounts given per 100g/100ml unless otherwise stated

Product	Brand	Calories kcal	Protein (g)	Carbohydrate (g)	Fat (g)	Dietary Fibre (g)
Shape Yogurts (St Ivel): see flavours						
Shapers (Boots): see flavours						
Shaschlik Sauce	Burgess	145	1.0	31.3	0.7	0.2
Shepherd's Pie per pack	Ross Birds Eye MenuMaster	114 275	5.2 11.0	12.0 35.0	5.2 11.0	0.5 n/a
Shepherd's Pie Cook In The Pot, as sold	Crosse & Blackwell	298	13.2	47.4	6.2	1.8
Shepherd's Pie Filling	Tyne Brand	111	8.2	5.5	6.4	n/a
Sherbet Dipper	Trebor Bassett	367	nil	90.5	nil	nil
Sherbet Fountain	Trebor Bassett	348	0.6	84.6	nil	0.1
Sherbet Fruits	Cravens	401	nil	83.9	8.4	nil
Sherbet Lemons, each	Trebor Bassett	23.0	n/a	6.1	n/a	n/a
Sherbet Orange, each	Trebor Bassett	23.0	n/a	6.1	n/a	n/a
Sherry *dry* *medium*		116 118	0.2 0.1	1.4 3.6	nil nil	nil nil

sweet		136	0.3	6.9	nil	nil
Sherry Gateau	McVitie's	329	2.8	28.8	22.6	0.1
Sherry Trifle, each	Birds Eye	180	2.5	16.5	7.5	n/a
Short Grain Rice	Whitworths	361	6.5	86.8	1.0	2.4
Shortbread						
Shortbread Fingers	Paterson's	498	5.9	63.9	26.1	1.9
Shortbread Mix, made up, per serving	Homepride Perfect	500	n/a	n/a	27.0	n/a
Shortbread Petticoat Tails	Paterson's	155	1.5	18.0	9.0	n/a
Shortbread Shapes	Paterson's	500	n/a	n/a	26.0	n/a
Shortcake Biscuits Dutch	Peek Frean Huntley & Palmer	464	5.4	67.0	21.2	1.8
Shortcake Snack	Cadbury	486	6.7	63.9	24.4	n/a
Shortcrust Pastry: see Pastry						
Shortcrust Pastry Mix, as sold	Homepride Perfect	492	8.0	55.0	26.0	nil

All amounts given per 100g/100ml unless otherwise stated

Product	Brand	Calories kcal	Protein (g)	Carbo-hydrate (g)	Fat (g)	Dietary Fibre (g)
Shredded Cabbage	Ross	16.0	1.4	5.5	0.1	3.2
Shredded Wheat		325	10.6	68.3	3.0	9.8
Shreddies		331	10.0	74.1	1.5	9.5
Shrimps, frozen, without shells canned, drained		73.0 94.0	16.5 20.8	nil nil	0.8 1.2	nil nil
Silverside, Sirloin: see Beef						
Silverskin Onions	Heinz	14.0	0.5	3.0	Tr	0.7
Singapore Curry Chinese Sauce Mix	Sharwood	296	4.3	67.5	2.8	n/a
Skate, fried in batter		199	17.9	4.9	12.1	0.2
Ski Fromage Frais, Salads, Yogurts (Eden Vale): see flavours						
Skimmed Milk: see Milk						
Skittles	Mars	384	0.3	91.6	4.4	n/a
Skull Truffles	Lyons	369	3.4	72.0	9.5	0.6
Sky Choc Bar, each	Wall's	210	2.5	19	15.0	n/a
Slender Plan Drinks, etc: see Carnation Slender Plan...						

Sliced Onions, dried	Whitworths	294	11.5	66.0	nil	16.6
Sliced Mushroom Ragu	Brooke Bond	77.0	1.9	11.8	2.7	n/a
Sliced Mushrooms, dried	Whitworths	188	32.3	3.4	3.0	15.4
Sliced Pepperoni Deep Pan Pizza	St Ivel	226	9.5	23.3	11.2	n/a
Sliced Poppadums	Sharwood	286	18.9	55.5	0.3	7.9
Smacks		386	8.0	89.6	2.0	3.0
Small Peas, canned	Batchelors	80.0	6.5	13.4	0.4	n/a
Smarties	Rowntree Mackintosh	455	5.5	74.5	17.1	n/a
Smatana, creamed	Raines	130	4.7	5.6	10.0	nil
Smoked Chicken & Bacon Ravioli	Dolmio	202	12.2	20.4	8.0	n/a
Smoked Fish: see *Cod, Haddock, etc*						
Smoked Ham, per slice	Delight	20.0	3.6	0.2	0.5	n/a
Smoked Ham & Mushroom Pizza						

All amounts given per 100g/100ml unless otherwise stated

Product	Brand	Calories kcal	Protein (g)	Carbohydrate (g)	Fat (g)	Dietary Fibre (g)
deep pan	McCain Pizza Perfection	183	10.7	27.0	4.3	n/a
pan bake	St Ivel	223	9.5	30.0	8.1	n/a
traditional	St Ivel	228	10.5	23.6	10.8	n/a
Smoked Mackerel in Fromage Frais	Lyons	339	10.7	7.5	29.7	n/a
Smoked Salmon in Fromage Frais	Lyons	373	9.7	2.7	36.0	n/a
Smokey Barbecue Sauce	Heinz	92.0	1.3	21.2	0.2	0.3
Smoky Cheddar with Paprika & Onion	St Ivel	415	25.7	1.7	33.7	n/a
Smooth Instant Chocolate Drink	Boots Shapers	353	16.0	57.0	8.4	4.7
Snickers	Mars	481	10.2	54.1	26.4	n/a
Snowballs	Tunnock's	388	3.9	47.0	21.8	n/a
Soda Water	Schweppes	nil	nil	nil	nil	nil
Sofrito Baked Beans	Crosse &					

	Blackwell	88.0	5.0	10.2	3.0	6.0
Soft Blackcurrant Flavour Gums, diabetic	Boots	234	7.9	81.0	0.3	nil
Soft Brown Bread	Hovis	224	8.4	41.3	2.1	4.6
Soft Cheese, medium fat	Delight	203	12.0	3.0	16.0	0.1
Soft Cheese with Fresh Garlic & Herbs, low fat	St Ivel Shape	132	11.6	2.8	8.4	n/a
Soft Cheese with Garlic & Herbs, low fat	Delight	145	11.0	3.0	10.0	0.1
Soft Cheese with Smoked Ham, low fat	St Ivel Shape	136	11.8	2.7	8.8	n/a
Soft Fruit Flavour Gums, diabetic	Boots	234	7.9	81.0	0.3	nil
Soft Wholemeal Bread	Nimble	238	12.6	37.6	4.1	6.6
Softgrain White Bread	Champion	230	7.5	45.0	1.5	3.8
Softgrain White Rolls	Champion	242	8.4	43.6	3.0	2.2
Softmints, each	Trebor Bassett	16.0	n/a	3.5	0.2	n/a

All amounts given per 100g/100ml unless otherwise stated

Product	Brand	Calories kcal	Protein (g)	Carbo-hydrate (g)	Fat (g)	Dietary Fibre (g)
Sole: *see Lemon Sole*						
Soup: *see flavours*						
Soup & Broth Mix	Whitworths	332	14.1	70.2	1.4	8.6
Sour Cream & Chives Dippits, per pack	Kavli	269	6.2	20.6	18.9	n/a
Southern Fried Chicken, each	Birds Eye	275	15.0	17.0	17.0	n/a
Soy & Chilli Sauce	Lea & Perrins	86.0	1.0	19.7	0.3	n/a
Soy & Five Spice Sauce	Lea & Perrins	98.0	1.4	21.7	0.5	n/a
Soy & Garlic Sauce	Lea & Perrins	88.0	0.9	19.8	0.6	n/a
Soy & Ginger Sauce	Lea & Perrins	96.0	1.5	21.4	0.4	n/a
Soy Chinese Pouring Sauce						
light	Sharwood	18.0	4.4	0.2	Tr	0.3
rich	Sharwood	48.0	4.6	7.5	Tr	0.3
Soy Sauce, dark, thick		64.0	8.7	8.3	nil	nil
Soya Banana Dessert	Granose	69.0	3.0	9.1	2.3	n/a
Soya Bean Curd: *see Tofu*						

Soya Bean Paste	Granose	140	11.0	5.5	7.5	n/a
Soya Beans, boiled		141	14.0	5.1	7.3	6.1
Soya Bran	Granose	100	14.0	35.0	3.0	35.0
Soya & Mushroom Burgers	Granose	250	11.5	23.6	12.8	n/a
Soya Chocolate Dessert	Granose	89.0	3.7	12.8	2.5	n/a
Soya Curd: *see Tofu*						
Soya Flour						
full fat		447	36.8	23.5	23.5	11.2
low fat		352	45.3	28.2	7.2	13.5
Soya Frankies	Granose	316	14.0	26.0	17.0	n/a
Soya Franks	Granose	265	9.3	3.2	23.9	n/a
Soya Margarine	Granose	745	0.1	0.1	82.0	n/a
Soya Milk, plain		32.0	2.9	0.8	1.9	nil
flavoured		40.0	2.8	3.6	1.7	nil
Soya Oil		899	Tr	nil	99.9	nil
Soya Strawberry Dessert	Granose	59.0	3.4	6.6	2.1	n/a
Soya Vanilla Dessert	Granose	79.0	3.1	11.7	2.2	n/a

All amounts given per 100g/100ml unless otherwise stated

Product	Brand	Calories kcal	Protein (g)	Carbohydrate (g)	Fat (g)	Dietary Fibre (g)
Soya Wurst, chicken flavour	Granose	59.0	3.4	6.6	2.1	n/a
Soya Yogurt: *see Yogurt*						
Soya Yogurts (Granose): *see flavours*						
Soyagen	Granose	501	17.4	53.7	24.0	n/a
Soyapro Beef	Granose	210	17.0	3.0	14.0	0.7
Soyapro Chicken	Granose	210	17.0	3.0	14.0	Tr
Soyapro Wieners	Granose	210	12.0	5.5	15.0	0.1
Spaghetti, cooked white wholemeal		104 / 113	3.6 / 4.7	22.2 / 23.2	0.7 / 0.9	1.2 / 3.5
Spaghetti, canned	Crosse & Blackwell / Heinz	65.0 / 65.0	1.8 / 1.7	13.5 / 14.1	0.4 / 0.2	0.1 / 0.4
Spaghetti Bolognese	Batchelors Microchef Snack	63.0	4.5	8.5	1.1	n/a
per pack	Birds Eye MenuMaster	375	19.0	56.0	10.0	n/a

per pack	Heinz Lunchbowl	113	5.1	13.5	4.3	1.1
	Mama Mia's	101	4.5	12.5	3.9	0.5
per pack canned	Heinz	90.0	3.3	13.8	2.4	0.5
low calorie	Findus Lean Cuisine	84.0	5.5	11.0	1.9	1.1
	Heinz Weight Watchers	88.0	5.5	11.9	2.0	1.0
Spaghetti Bolognese Casserole Sauce Mix						
with mushrooms	Colman's	328	11.0	n/a	1.3	n/a
with peppers	Colman's	329	9.6	n/a	1.3	n/a
Spaghetti Bolognese Sauce						
with mushrooms	Campbell's	62.0	2.7	9.4	1.5	0.1
	Campbell's	66.0	2.6	10.4	1.6	0.1
with onions & garlic	Campbell's	66.0	2.6	10.3	106	0.2
Spaghetti Hoops						
no added sugar	Heinz	66.0	1.9	14.1	0.2	0.7
	Heinz Weight Watchers	51.0	1.7	10.5	0.2	0.4
Spaghetti Sauce Mix	Knorr	339	7.9	65.5	6.8	5.7
Spaghetti Shapes	Heinz Haunted					

All amounts given per 100g/100ml unless otherwise stated

Product	Brand	Calories kcal	Protein (g)	Carbo-hydrate (g)	Fat (g)	Dietary Fibre (g)
	House	72.0	2.2	16.2	0.3	0.7
	Heinz Noodle Doodles	630	1.5	13.5	0.3	0.7
Spaghetti with Sausages in Tomato Sauce	Heinz	119	3.4	14.5	5.3	0.6
Spanish Lentil Soup	Rakusen	27.0	2.7	4.7	0.5	n/a
Spanish Paella Stir Fry	Ross	80.0	5.2	12.4	1.4	0.7
Spare Rib Casserole Sauce	Crosse & Blackwell	99.0	1.5	19.4	1.2	0.6
Sparkles, orange/lemon, each	Wall's	30.0	Tr	8.0	Tr	n/a
Spearmint Chewing Gum (Wrigley): see Chewing Gum						
Special Chinese Rice	Sharwood	364	8.4	72.1	3.5	3.0
Special K		377	15.3	81.7	1.0	2.0
Special Recipe Muesli	Jordans	364	10.6	57.9	2.9	9.0
Special Reserve Premium Cider	HP Bulmer	52.0	n/a	n/a	n/a	n/a

Special Rice Mix	Ross	59.0	2.6	13.5	0.4	2.0
Spiced Basmati Rice	Sharwood	360	9.1	75.4	1.0	1.5
Spiced Fruit Chutney	Baxters	131	0.6	34.1	Tr	1.1
Spiced Vegetable Chutney	Sharwood	161	1.0	40.0	0.4	1.7
Spicy Apple Lunchbar	Boots Shapers	409	8.3	49.0	20.0	n/a
Spicy Apple Microbake Mix, made up, per serving	Homepride	261	3.0	47.5	6.0	n/a
Spicy Barbecue Sauce	Colman's	59.0	0.8	n/a	0.2	n/a
Spicy Bean Salad	Batchelors	129	7.0	23.8	1.3	n/a
Spicy Beef & Rice Soup	Heinz Weight Watchers	27.0	1.1	4.4	0.5	0.2
Spicy Beef & Tomato Soup	Heinz	43.0	2.2	7.0	0.7	0.7
Spicy Beef French Bread Pizza	Findus Lean Cuisine	177	9.0	24.6	4.7	1.6
Spicy Beef Luxury Pizza, each	Birds Eye Gino Ginelli	580	30.0	80.0	18.0	n/a
Spicy Beef Stew, canned	Tyne Brand	106	7.5	8.1	5.1	n/a

All amounts given per 100g/100ml unless otherwise stated

Product	Brand	Calories kcal	Protein (g)	Carbo-hydrate (g)	Fat (g)	Dietary Fibre (g)
Spicy Bombay Fish Curry	Findus Dinner Supreme	117	5.9	12.3	5.3	1.0
Spicy Chicken & Rice Soup low calorie	Heinz Heinz Weight Watchers	59.0	4.2	7.8	1.2	0.8
	Heinz Weight Watchers	27.0	1.9	4.1	0.3	0.3
Spicy Chicken Creole with Rice	Findus Lean Cuisine	100	7.0	14.9	1.4	1.3
Spicy Chicken Mexican Chilli Sauce	Homepride	80.0	1.0	17.0	n/a	n/a
Spicy Parsnip Soup	Baxters	20.0	2.3	5.4	2.2	1.4
Spicy Pepper Sauce	Heinz	84.0	1.6	18.2	0.5	0.1
Spicy Pepperoni Pizza	McVitie's	194	8.5	26.3	6.7	1.5
Spicy Rice Salad	Eden Vale	176	2.4	18.2	10.9	n/a
Spicy Sauce	Branston	115	1.0	23.9	0.7	1.3
Spicy Tomato Ragu	Brooke Bond	84.0	2.0	13.0	3.0	n/a
Spicy Tomato Sauce	HP	121	1.6	26.5	1.0	n/a
Spinach, raw		25.0	2.8	1.6	0.8	2.1

boiled		19.0	2.2	0.8	0.8		2.1
frozen, boiled		21.0	3.1	0.5	0.8		2.1
Spira	Cadbury	520	7.7	58.7	29.9	nil	n/a
Spiral Oven Fries	McCain	196	2.0	31.4	7.8	nil	n/a
Spirits, 40% volume *(mean of brandy gin, rum, whisky)*		222	Tr	Tr		nil	nil
Split Peas, dried, boiled		126	8.3	22.7	0.9		2.7
Sponge Cake		459	6.4	52.4	26.3	0.9	
fatless		294	10.1	53.0	6.1	0.9	
jam filled		302	4.2	64.2	4.9	1.8	
with butter icing		490	4.5	52.4	30.6	0.6	
Sponge Cake Mixes: see flavours							
Sponge Finger Biscuits	Huntley & Palmer	400	7.4	90.6	4.0	0.5	
Sponge Pudding *(see also flavours)*		340	5.8	45.3	16.3	1.1	
Sport Biscuits	McVitie's	516	6.4	62.9	26.5	1.7	
Spotted Dick	McVitie's	357	5.7	51.2	15.0	2.3	
	Mr Kipling	349	5.0	48.8	16.0	n/a	

All amounts given per 100g/100ml unless otherwise stated

Product	Brand	Calories kcal	Protein (g)	Carbo-hydrate (g)	Fat (g)	Dietary Fibre (g)
Spotted Dick Microbake Mix, made up, per serving	Homepride	237	4.0	38.0	7.0	n/a
Spreads, Dairy, Low Fat, etc: see brands/flavours						
Spring Greens, raw		33.0	3.0	3.1	1.0	3.4
boiled		20.0	1.9	1.6	0.7	0.7
Spring Onion Crisps	Golden Wonder	153	2.0	12.6	10.5	n/a
Spring Onions, bulbs & tops, raw		23.0	2.0	3.0	0.5	1.5
Spring Vegetable Soup	Heinz	34.0	1.0	7.6	Tr	0.9
Sprouts: see Brussels Sprouts						
Squash: see Courgettes						
Start		355	7.9	81.7	1.7	5.7
Steak: see Beef						
Steak & Ale Pie	Fray Bentos	210	8.6	15.9	12.9	n/a
Steak & Ale Pie with Onion Filling	Fray Bentos	122	9.9	4.0	7.5	n/a
Steak & Ale Pudding	Fray Bentos	220	7.5	19.0	12.0	n/a

Steak & Kidney Pancakes	Findus	151	6.2	2.25	4.0	1.0
Steak & Kidney Pie, individual pastry top only		323	9.1	25.6	21.2	0.9
		286	15.2	15.9	18.4	0.6
	Ross Golden Choice	289	7.1	24.3	18.6	1.0
	Ross Hungryman	248	9.7	18.3	15.1	0.8
each	Birds Eye Homebake	370	13.0	32.0	22.0	n/a
canned, 213g	Fray Bentos	202	9.7	15.0	12.0	n/a
canned, 425g	Fray Bentos	197	9.3	14.6	11.6	n/a
Steak & Kidney Pie Platter, per pack	Birds Eye MenuMaster	515	25.0	60.0	21.0	n/a
Steak & Kidney Pie Filling	Fray Bentos	123	9.7	3.3	8.0	n/a
Steak & Kidney Pudding						
213g	Fray Bentos	204	8.7	20.1	10.3	n/a
425g	Fray Bentos	214	8.8	20.2	11.5	n/a
Steak & Mushroom Pie Filling	Fray Bentos	106	9.4	4.3	5.8	n/a
Steak & Vegetable Pie, 213g	Fray Bentos	175	6.7	14.9	10.3	n/a

All amounts given per 100g/100ml unless otherwise stated

Product	Brand	Calories kcal	Protein (g)	Carbo-hydrate (g)	Fat (g)	Dietary Fibre (g)
425g	Fray Bentos	185	6.3	16.8	10.7	n/a
Steak & Vegetable Pie Filling	Fray Bentos	115	7.0	6.0	10.5	n/a
Steak & Vegetable Pudding	Fray Bentos	215	6.0	21.0	12.5	n/a
Stew: see flavours						
Stewed Steak with Gravy, canned		176	14.8	1.0	1.25	Tr
Still Lemonade	Del Monte Fruit Burst	42.0	0.2	10.6	Tr	n/a
Stilton & Celery Soup	Baxters	83.0	3.5	4.3	5.4	0.2
Stilton, blue	St Ivel	411	22.7	0.1	35.5	nil
white		360	19.9	0.2	31.3	nil
Stir Fry Indian Mild Curry Rice	Uncle Ben's	207	3.3	36.1	5.5	n/a
Stir Fry Chinese Style Rice	Uncle Ben's	164	3.2	29.7	4.4	n/a
Stock Cubes: see flavours						
Stoneground Wholemeal Baps, each	Allinson	139	5.9	22.4	2.9	3.6

Stoneground Wholemeal Bread 100% with organic flour	Hovis	213	9.5	37.3	2.3	6.7
	Allinson	219	9.7	38.5	3.0	6.5
	Hovis	231	9.8	40.0	2.9	7.1
Stork Light Blend Spread	Van Den Berghs	542	0.1	0.4	60.0	n/a
Stork Margarine	Van Den Berghs	732	0.1	0.4	81.0	n/a
Special Blend	Van Den Berghs	733	0.1	0.4	81.0	n/a
Stout, bottled		37.0	0.3	4.2	Tr	nil
extra		39.0	0.3	2.1	Tr	nil
Straw Mushroom: see Mushrooms						
Strawberries, raw		27.0	0.8	6.0	0.1	1.1
canned in syrup		65.0	0.5	16.9	Tr	0.7
Strawberries & Cream Frousse	Ski	161	4.7	18.5	8.1	n/a
Strawberry & Apple Fruit Pie	Lyons	370	3.0	58.8	15.2	1.5
Strawberry & Apple Juice	Copella	39.0	n/a	10.1	nil	Tr
Strawberry & Blackberry Fruit on Bottom Yogurt	Ski	86.0	4.8	16.2	0.7	n/a

All amounts given per 100g/100ml unless otherwise stated

Product	Brand	Calories kcal	Protein (g)	Carbo-hydrate (g)	Fat (g)	Dietary Fibre (g)
Strawberry & Coconut Tropical Yogurt	St Ivel Shape	42.0	4.7	5.7	0.1	n/a
Strawberry & Cream Dairy Ice Cream	Boots Shapers	102	2.7	15.0	3.9	Tr
Strawberry & Cream Mivvi, each	Lyons Maid	87.0	1.1	13.8	2.8	n/a
Strawberry & Guava Soya Dessert	Granose	94.0	1.3	14.5	3.8	n/a
Strawberry & Peach Real Fruit Le Yogurt, stirred, low fat	Chambourcy	89.0	5.0	16.7	0.6	Tr
Strawberry & Redcurrant Bio Fruit on Bottom Yogurt	Ski	106	5.4	15.9	2.8	n/a
Strawberry & Vanilla Fromage Frais	St Ivel Shape	50.0	6.8	5.7	0.2	n/a
Strawberry & Vanilla Yogurt diet, Greek style low calorie	Boots Shapers	89.0	4.8	7.9	4.2	Tr
	St Ivel Shape	41.0	4.7	5.6	0.1	n/a

thick & creamy	Boots	86.0	4.8	16.2	0.7	n/a
Strawberry & Wild Strawberry Fruit on Bottom Yogurt	Ski	86.0	4.8	16.2	0.7	n/a
Strawberry Carob Coated Fruit Bar, each	Granose	170	3.3	31.5	3.4	3.4
Strawberry Blancmange	Brown & Polson	330	0.4	87.4	0.1	n/a
Strawberry Bonbons, each	Trebor Bassett	27.0	n/a	5.9	0.4	n/a
Strawberry Carmelle Mix made up, per serving	Homepride Classic	189	5.5	26.0	7.0	n/a
Strawberry Cheesecake	Chambourcy	244	6.0	32.5	10.0	1.1
	Eden Vale	261	2.8	38.8	11.6	n/a
	McVitie's	324	4.7	30.0	20.7	0.4
	Young's	240	5.5	2.55	13.1	0.5
individual						
Strawberry Cheesecake Mix, made up	Lyons Tetley	250	4.1	30.0	12.0	n/a
Strawberry Cornetto, each	Wall's	190	2.5	28.0	8.0	n/a
Strawberry Cream Cake	McVitie's	274	2.9	36.2	13.5	1.0

All amounts given per 100g/100ml unless otherwise stated

Product	Brand	Calories kcal	Protein (g)	Carbo-hydrate (g)	Fat (g)	Dietary Fibre (g)
Strawberry Creme De Creme Ice Cream Cup	Lyons Maid	174	2.3	26.0	7.2	n/a
Strawberry Creme Sundae Yogurt	St Ivel Shape	41.0	4.7	5.6	0.1	n/a
Strawberry Crusha	Burgess	112	Tr	27.4	nil	nil
Strawberry Dairy Dessert	St Ivel Fiendish Feet	91.0	4.9	16.1	1.2	n/a
Strawberry Dairy Ice Cream	Lyons Maid Napoli	75.0	1.5	11.3	3.0	n/a
Strawberry Devonshire Cheesecake	St Ivel	250	6.3	26.5	140	n/a
Strawberry Fancies	Lyons	498	4.9	55.5	30.0	0.3
Strawberry Flavour Dessert Mix, diabetic	Boots	131	3.1	15.2	6.4	Tr
Strawberry Fool Mix, made up	Lyons Tetley	153	3.6	20.8	5.9	n/a
Strawberry Fresta	Wall's	80.0	2.0	14.0	2.0	n/a
Strawberry Fromage Frais	Ski	137	6.7	13.7	6.5	n/a

each / low calorie						
Strawberry Fruit Fool	Birds Eye Healthy Options	145	4.0	22.0	5.0	n/a
	Diet Ski	69.0	8.2	6.0	1.5	n/a
	St Ivel Shape	49.0	6.8	5.3	0.2	n/a
Strawberry Fruit Swirl Yogurt	Boots Shapers	119	2.4	5.7	9.8	n/a
	Gold Ski	109	4.6	15.8	3.5	0.4
Strawberry Gateau Individual	McVitie's	277	2.3	30.4	16.4	n/a
	St Ivel	236	2.2	24.7	14.9	0.4
Strawberry Jam diabetic	Applefords	113	0.1	20.5	Tr	n/a
	Boots	163	0.3	64.0	nil	1.6
reduced sugar	Dietade	248	0.2	65.8	n/a	n/a
	Heinz Weight Watchers	125	0.4	33.0	Tr	1.1
Strawberry Jam Sponge Pudding	Heinz	299	2.6	49.8	9.9	0.8
Strawberry Jelly Crystals	Dietade	7.0	1.5	0.3	n/a	n/a
Strawberry Jelly, ready to eat	Rowntree	67.0	0.1	16.7	Tr	0.5
Strawberry Monster Mousse	St Ivel Fiendish Feet	63.0	2.2	10.9	1.5	n/a

All amounts given per 100g/100ml unless otherwise stated

Product	Brand	Calories kcal	Protein (g)	Carbo-hydrate (g)	Fat (g)	Dietary Fibre (g)
Strawberry Nesquik made up with whole milk	Nestlé	391	nil	96.7	0.5	nil
with semi-skimmed milk	Nestlé	168	6.8	18.8	3.7	n/a
	Nestlé	131	6.8	18.8	3.7	n/a
ready to drink	Nestlé	68.0	3.2	10.0	1.7	nil
Strawberry Pavlova	McVitie's	330	2.3	32.7	21.1	Tr
Strawberry Preserve	Baxters	200	Tr	53.0	Tr	1.4
Strawberry Puff Slices	Lyons	506	3.0	48.0	34.9	1.1
Strawberry Sherbets, each	Trebor Bassett	23.0	n/a	6.1	n/a	n/a
Strawberry Ski Bar Frozen Yogurt	Ski	258	4.3	32.7	13.1	n/a
Strawberry Ski Cone, frozen	Ski	242	14.0	34.8	6.2	n/a
Strawberry Soya Yogurt	Granose	69.0	3.0	11.4	1.6	n/a
Strawberry Split, each	Wall's	79.0	1.0	13.0	2.5	n/a
Strawberry Split Yogurt	Gold Ski	130	4.9	20.1	3.9	n/a
Strawberry Supermousse, each	Birds Eye	110	2.0	19.5	3.2	n/a

Strawberry Supreme	Eden Vale	118	2.8	20.2	3.5	n/a
Strawberry Tartlets, each	Mr Kipling	164	2.1	24.9	6.9	n/a
Strawberry Trembler	St Ivel Fiendish Feet	72.0	2.7	15.3	0.4	n/a
Strawberry Trifle	Eden Vale	160	2.4	25.0	6.3	n/a
	St Ivel	143	1.2	23.0	5.7	n/a
	Young's	142	1.4	26.6	3.7	0.2
Strawberry Vanilla Ice Cream	Delight	157	3.7	23.9	5.8	nil
Strawberry Yogurt	Gold Ski	111	5.3	17.1	2.8	nil
	St Ivel Real	89.0	5.0	15.0	1.0	nil
extrafruit	Ski	84.0	4.2	16.3	0.7	nil
French style	St Ivel Shape	40.0	4.8	5.3	0.1	nil
fruit on bottom	Ski	89.0	4.8	16.8	0.7	nil
Greek style	Boots	145	4.8	18.0	8.6	nil
lightly whipped	St Ivel Prize	135	4.3	15.2	6.4	nil
long life	St Ivel Prize	62.0	3.5	12.5	0.1	nil
low calorie	Boots Shapers	43.0	4.4	6.5	0.1	0.2
	St Ivel Shape	41.0	4.7	5.6	0.1	nil
low fat	Boots	96.0	4.6	18.0	1.1	nil
	Diet Ski	35.0	3.9	4.6	0.2	nil

All amounts given per 100g/100ml unless otherwise stated

Product	Brand	Calories kcal	Protein (g)	Carbo-hydrate (g)	Fat (g)	Dietary Fibre (g)
pasteurised, very low fat twinpot	Dairy Crest	86.0	3.8	18.0	0.4	nil
	St Ivel Shape	56.0	4.3	8.3	0.9	nil
Strawberry Yogurt Drink	Ski Cool	71.0	3.1	15.0	0.3	n/a
Strawberry Yogurt Mousse Slice	Boots Shapers	147	3.2	22.0	1.0	1.0
Strike Cola	Barr	33.0	n/a	n/a	n/a	n/a
diet	Barr	1.1	n/a	n/a	n/a	n/a
Stringfellows Fast Fry Chips	McCain	123	2.9	25.0	3.2	n/a
Stringfellows Oven Chips	McCain	180	2.7	26.0	7.2	n/a
Strollers	Cadbury	460	5.6	65.4	21.6	n/a
Strong Ale		72.0	0.7	6.1	Tr	nil
Strongbow Cider bottle/can	HP Bulmer	36.0	n/a	n/a	n/a	n/a
draught	HP Bulmer	35.0	n/a	n/a	n/a	n/a
1080	HP Bulmer	49.0	n/a	n/a	n/a	n/a
super	HP Bulmer	52.0	n/a	n/a	n/a	n/a
LA	HP Bulmer	16.0	n/a	n/a	n/a	n/a

Stuffed Pork Roll	Tyne Brand	153	10.75	9.6	8.3	n/a
Stuffed Turkey Roll	Tyne Brand	144	11.7	7.8	7.6	n/a
Stuffing Mixes: see flavours						
Suet, shredded		826	Tr	12.1	86.7	0.5
Sugar: see Caster, Granulated, etc						
Sugar Puffs		324	5.9	84.5	0.8	3.2
Sugared Almonds, original	Cravens	430	6.4	72.9	14.2	5.8
Sultana & Apple Crunch	Mornflake	390	12.0	60.0	13.0	14.0
Sultana & Apple Slices	Lyons	398	3.9	64.4	15.6	2.0
Sultana & Cherry Cake	Lyons	335	4.4	55.3	12.3	2.5
Sultana & Ginger Wholemeal Cake Mix	Granose	387	12.5	52.4	10.7	n/a
Sultana & Hazelnut Crunch 'n' Slim	Crookes Healthcare	415	10.5	56.0	18.0	1.1
Sultana & Nut Cookies	Boots	495	5.7	61.0	27.0	2.8
Sultana & Syrup Loaf	Sunblest	279	9.0	56.8	1.7	3.4

All amounts given per 100g/100ml unless otherwise stated

Product	Brand	Calories kcal	Protein (g)	Carbo-hydrate (g)	Fat (g)	Dietary Fibre (g)
Sultana & Syrup Pancakes	Sunblest	275	5.8	48.9	6.2	2.2
Sultana Bran		303	8.5	67.8	1.6	10.0
Sultana Cake	Lyons	340	4.5	56.4	12.3	3.3
Sultana Scones	Mothers Pride	333	7.6	50.8	10.5	2.7
Sultanas		275	2.7	69.4	0.4	2.0
Summer County Dairy Spread	Van Den Berghs	542	0.1	0.4	60.0	n/a
Summer Orchard	Kellogg's	330	9.0	62.0	5.0	8.0
Summerfruits Fruit on Bottom Yogurt bio	Ski Ski	95.0 104	4.8 5.4	18.4 15.2	0.7 2.8	n/a n/a
Summerfruits Split Yogurt	Gold Ski	115	4.9	16.0	3.9	n/a
Sunblest Bread, etc (Allied Bakeries): see flavours						
Sunflower Margarine	Rakusen Vitalite	740 730	n/a 0.2	n/a 1.3	82.0 80.0	n/a nil
Sunflower Seed Oil		899	Tr	nil	99.9	nil
Sunflower/Sesame Roast	Granose	488	19.9	33.2	30.6	n/a

Sunflower Spread reduced fat	St Ivel Shape Vitalite	366 540	6.0 0.2	3.0 1.3	36.8 59.0	n/a nil
Super Deluxe Deep Pan Pizza	McCain Pizza Perfection	195	9.9	28.0	5.5	n/a
Supermousse Tub Dessert (Birds Eye): *see flavours*						
Supernoodles (Batchelors): *see flavours*						
Superwhip	Birds Eye	126	1.4	9.5	9.0	n/a
Supreme (Eden Vale): *see flavours*						
Supreme Cook-In-Sauce	Homepride	72.0	1.0	9.0	n/a	n/a
Swede, boiled		11.0	0.3	2.3	0.1	0.7
Sweet & Sour Bistro Break	HP	112	5.8	18.6	1.6	1.5
Sweet & Sour Casserole Recipe Sauce	Knorr	58.0	0.9	14.5	Tr	n/a
Sweet & Sour Chicken	Vesta	108	2.8	22.8	1.2	n/a
Sweet & Sour Chicken with Rice, per pack	Birds Eye MenuMaster	385	21.0	73.0	3.0	n/a
Sweet & Sour Cook-In-Sauce	Homepride	58.0	0.4	13.1	n/a	n/a

All amounts given per 100g/100ml unless otherwise stated

Product	Brand	Calories kcal	Protein (g)	Carbo-hydrate (g)	Fat (g)	Dietary Fibre (g)
Sweet & Sour Pork Cook In The Pot Microwave Mix, as sold	Crosse & Blackwell	371	2.7	81.5	3.1	0.4
Sweet & Sour Pork Stir Fry Cook In The Pot Dry Mix, as sold	Crosse & Blackwell	386	7.1	61.8	12.3	1.8
Sweet & Sour Sauce	Burgess	150	0.6	35.2	Tr	0.2
	HP	143	0.5	31.8	1.4	n/a
Sweet & Sour Sauce & Vegetable Stir Fry	Uncle Ben's	94.0	0.4	23.2	Tr	n/a
Sweet & Sour Sauce Mix, dry, as sold	Colman's	305	7.4	n/a	0.8	n/a
jar	Colman's	71.0	0.8	n/a	Tr	n/a
Sweet & Sour Stir Fry Sauce	Sharwood	148	0.2	39.0	0.1	n/a
	Uncle Ben's	165	0.6	39.4	0.5	n/a
Sweet & Sour Vegetable Soup	Baxters	20.0	0.5	4.9	0.1	0.6
Sweet Corn, Peas & Carrots, 1oz/28g	Birds Eye	17.0	1.0	3.0	0.5	n/a

Sweet Orange Marmalade	Baxters	200	Tr	53.0	Tr	0.8
Sweet Peanuts, each	Trebor Bassett	26.0	n/a	4.8	0.7	Tr
Sweet Pepper Pasta Choice Dry Mix, as sold	Crosse & Blackwell	363	12.4	69.7	3.8	2.4
Sweet Pickle	Burgess	167	0.9	39.3	Tr	1.9
Sweet Potato, boiled		84.0	1.1	20.5	0.3	2.3
Sweetbread, lamb, fried		230	19.4	5.6	14.6	0.1
Sweetcorn						
baby, fresh/frozen, boiled		24.0	2.5	2.7	0.4	2.0
baby, canned		23.0	2.9	2.0	0.4	1.5
kernels, boiled		111	4.2	19.6	2.3	2.2
kernels, canned		122	2.9	26.6	1.2	1.4
on-the-cob, boiled		66.0	2.5	11.6	1.4	1.3
Swiss Gateau	Cadbury	403	5.5	60.3	17.2	n/a
Swiss Rolls: *see also flavours*						
Swiss Rolls, chocolate, individual		337	4.3	58.1	11.3	N
Swiss Style Chocolate Cake Mix, made up, per serving	Green's	228	2.0	31.0	12.0	n/a

All amounts given per 100g/100ml unless otherwise stated

Product	Brand	Calories kcal	Protein (g)	Carbo-hydrate (g)	Fat (g)	Dietary Fibre (g)
Syrup, Golden		298	0.3	79.0	nil	nil
Syrup Microbake Mix, made up, per serving	Homepride	271	3.0	44.0	9.0	n/a
Syrup Sponge Pudding Mix, made up, per serving	Homepride Perfect	294	4.5	56.5	5.5	nil
Szechuan Chilli Sauce & Vegetable Stir Fry	Uncle Ben's	85.0	0.9	10.5	4.3	n/a
Szechuan Pork with Vegetable Chow Mein	Heinz	117	5.6	11.3	5.5	0.8
Szechuan Spicy Pork Microwave Meal	Sharwood	147	7.6	20.3	3.7	1.3
Szechuan Spicy Tomato Cook-In-Sauce	Homepride	104	0.9	19.4	n/a	n/a

T

Table Water Biscuits	McVitie's	436	9.3	76.7	9.1	3.2
Taco Sauce, hot	Old El Paso	43.0	n/a	n/a	n/a	n/a
mild	Old El Paso	41.0	n/a	n/a	n/a	n/a
Taco Shells	Old El Paso	463	n/a	n/a	n/a	n/a
Tagliatelle Bianche	Dolmio	141	4.9	29.1	1.4	n/a
Tagliatelle Carbonara	Boots Shapers	99.0	4.9	6.6	6.1	1.6
Tagliatelle Garlic & Herbs	Dolmio	149	5.6	28.8	1.3	n/a
Tahini Paste		607	18.5	0.9	58.9	8.0
Tandoori Chicken Masala	Findus Dinner Supreme	147	5.4	19.0	6.0	1.0
Tandoori Classic Curry Sauce	Homepride	70.0	1.4	8.5	n/a	n/a

All amounts given per 100g/100ml unless otherwise stated

Product	Brand	Calories kcal	Protein (g)	Carbohydrate (g)	Fat (g)	Dietary Fibre (g)
Tandoori Curry Paste	Sharwood	241	5.5	10.4	19.7	4.6
Tandoori Curry Sauce Mix, as sold	Sharwood	224	9.4	33.6	6.7	n/a
Tandoori Fried Savoury Rice	Batchelors	365	11.1	67.4	7.5	n/a
Tandoori Sauce	HP	102	1.2	21.7	1.1	n/a
Tangerine Flavour Jelly Crystals, diabetic	Boots	348	71.0	16.0	Tr	nil
Tangerines, flesh only		35.0	1.0	18.0	1.5	1.3
Tangle Twister, each	Wall's	85.0	0.6	n/a	Tr	n/a
Tangy Apricot Lunchbar	Boots Shapers	409	8.3	49.0	20.0	n/a
Tangy Barbecue Sauce	Colman's	58.0	0.6	n/a	Tr	n/a
Tangy Fruit Fancies, each	Mr Kipling	104	0.7	20.2	2.8	n/a
Tangy Pickle Spread	Heinz Ploughman's	130	0.7	31.8	Tr	1.3
Tapioca, creamed	Ambrosia	83.0	2.9	13.8	1.8	n/a
Taramasalata		446	3.2	4.1	46.4	N

Tartare Sauce	Burgess	288	1.4	19.5	21.9	0.3
	Colman's	309	6.6	n/a	1.4	n/a
Tastex	Granose	208	38.0	15.0	Tr	n/a
Teacakes	Tunnock's	413	5.2	61.0	18.1	n/a
Teacakes, toasted		329	8.9	58.3	8.3	N
Tea Crackers	Rakusen	347	9.5	80.0	1.0	3.0
Tea Matzos	Rakusen	347	9.5	80.0	1.0	3.0
Tender Bits	Granose	79.0	13.5	5.7	0.4	0.2
Tendercrisp Corn	Green Giant	52.0	n/a	n/a	nil	n/a
Teriyaki Stir Fry Sauce	Sharwood	74.0	0.7	16.2	0.8	0.4
Texas Barbecue Cook-In-Sauce	Homepride	71.0	1.4	14.1	n/a	n/a
Thai Curry Sauce & Vegetables Stir Fry	Uncle Ben's	84.0	1.0	10.7	4.1	n/a
Thai Hot Chicken Curry Microwave Meal	Sharwood	137	5.5	17.0	5.0	1.3

All amounts given per 100g/100ml unless otherwise stated

Product	Brand	Calories kcal	Protein (g)	Carbohydrate (g)	Fat (g)	Dietary Fibre (g)
Thai Hot Curry Paste	Sharwood	218	4.7	8.5	18.4	6.7
Thai Hot Curry Sauce	Sharwood	107	2.3	7.2	7.8	2.4
Thai Sauce For Rice	Sharwood	44.0	1.7	8.6	0.3	1.1
Thick Country Vegetable with Ham Soup	Heinz	55.0	2.0	6.6	2.3	1.2
Thick Winter Soup	Rakusen	40.0	1.9	7.1	0.8	n/a
Thousand Island Dressing	Burgess	586	1.8	12.6	58.3	Tr
	Flora	53.0	Tr	1.5	5.4	n/a
	Heinz All Seasons	286	1.0	20.0	22.4	0.3
	Kraft	393	1.0	14.0	37.0	n/a
fat free	Kraft	98.0	0.6	25.5	Tr	n/a
Thousand Island Dip	Burgess	571	2.4	13.1	56.0	0.4
Thousand Island Prawnnaise	Lyons	451	5.7	3.3	46.9	n/a
Thread Noodles	Sharwood	323	11.5	69.2	1.9	3.4
Three Fruits Marmalade	Baxters	200	Tr	53.0	Tr	0.1
Tiffin	Cadbury	480	6.3	64.3	23.7	n/a

Tiger Prawns, cooked & peeled	Lyons	53.0	12.0	nil	0.6	n/a
Tigertots	Rowntree Mackintosh	376	1.7	85.2	5.5	n/a
Tikka Classic Curry Sauce	Homepride	80.0	2.2	8.9	n/a	n/a
Tikka Curry Paste	Sharwood	158	1.4	7.0	12.6	4.8
Tikka Dippits, per pack	Kavli	265	5.6	21.9	18.2	n/a
Tikka Masala Classic Curry Sauce	Homepride	94.0	2.2	11.8	n/a	n/a
Tikka Masala Curry Sauce, canned	Sharwood	99.0	3.0	8.4	5.8	2.3
Tikka Prawnmaise Light	Lyons	218	5.2	6.1	19.3	n/a
Tip Top (Nestlé): see Cream, imitation						
Tiramisu	McVitie's	324	3.0	27.7	22.5	0.3
Tizer	Barr	41.0	n/a	n/a	n/a	n/a
diet	Barr	0.5	n/a	n/a	n/a	n/a
Toad In The Hole	Findus	233	8.6	2.05	13.5	1.0

All amounts given per 100g/100ml unless otherwise stated

Product	Brand	Calories kcal	Protein (g)	Carbo-hydrate (g)	Fat (g)	Dietary Fibre (g)
Toast: see Bread						
Toast Toppers (Heinz): see flavours						
Toasted Oat Crunchy	Mornflake	338	11.0	52.0	11.0	11.0
Toasted Teacakes	Trebor Bassett	452	3.4	2.8	26.0	9.5
Toffee & Apple Yogurt, low fat	Boots	97.0	4.7	18.0	1.2	n/a
Toffee & Mallow Easter Egg, each	Rowntree Mackintosh	120	1.4	18.2	5.1	n/a
Toffee & Mixed Nuts Thick & Creamy Yogurt	Boots	131	5.1	20.0	4.0	n/a
Toffee Apple Dairy Dessert	St Ivel Fiendish Feet	91.0	4.9	16.1	1.2	n/a
Toffee Bon Bons, each	Trebor Bassett	27.0	n/a	5.9	0.4	n/a
Toffee Crisp	Rowntree Mackintosh	507	5.2	62.4	28.0	n/a
Toffee Crumble Mivvi, each	Lyons Maid	153	1.8	17.3	9.0	n/a
Toffee Crusha	Burgess	175	nil	43.1	nil	nil

Toffee Cup Cakes	Lyons	391	3.3	67.7	13.8	0.5
Toffee Filled Easter Egg, each	Rowntree Mackintosh	100	0.7	14.3	4.8	n/a
Toffee Freddie Mix, made up, per serving	Homepride	55.0	1.0	9.0	1.5	n/a
Toffee Fudge Ice Cream	Wall's Gino Ginelli Tub	110	2.0	16.0	4.5	n/a
Toffee Fudge Supermousse, each	Birds Eye	172	2.6	22.0	8.4	n/a
Toffee Microbake Mix, made up, per serving	Homepride	212	3.0	36.0	n/a	n/a
Toffee Monster Mousse	St Ivel Fiendish Feet	67.0	2.1	11.8	1.6	n/a
Toffee YoYo	McVitie's	476	5.3	66.9	20.9	1.0
Toffees, diabetic	Boots	322	1.3	78.0	14.0	Tr
Toffees, mixed		430	2.1	71.1	17.2	nil
Toffo, assorted	Rowntree Mackintosh	453	2.3	73.2	18.8	n/a

All amounts given per 100g/100ml unless otherwise stated

Product	Brand	Calories kcal	Protein (g)	Carbohydrate (g)	Fat (g)	Dietary Fibre (g)
plain	Rowntree Mackintosh	452	2.3	74.3	18.2	n/a
mint	Rowntree Mackintosh	432	2.3	77.7	14.6	n/a
Tofu (soya bean curd)						
steamed		73.0	8.1	0.7	4.2	N
steamed, fried		261	23.5	2.0	17.7	N
Tomato & Cheese Pizza	McVitie's	186	8.0	27.1	5.9	1.9
Tomato & Chilli Dip	Burgess	486	2.8	12.9	46.3	0.5
Tomato & Courgette Chutney	Baxters	110	0.7	28.4	0.1	0.6
	Sharwood	80.0	0.8	18.7	0.4	0.9
Tomato & Green Pepper soup	Heinz Spicy Soups	45.0	1.0	8.5	0.8	0.2
Tomato & Herb Oatsters	Jordans	401	11.7	58.5	15.0	7.0
Tomato & Lentil Soup	Heinz Whole Soups	57.0	2.8	11.2	0.1	1.5
Tomato & Onion Casserole Recipe Sauce	Knorr	71.0	1.3	10.9	2.8	n/a

Tomato & Onion Cook-In-Sauce	Homepride	51.0	1.1	10.3	n/a	n/a
Tomato & Onion Mello 'n' Mild	Colman's	128	3.1	n/a	2.1	n/a
Tomato & Onion Soup, condensed	Campbell's	46.0	1.2	10.3	nil	0.3
Tomato & Onion Spread	Heinz	210	1.7	24.3	11.8	1.4
Tomato & Orange Soup	Baxters	40.0	1.0	8.5	0.5	0.3
Tomato & Oregano Dip & Snack	Boots Shapers	483	17.9	61.2	20.0	22.8
Tomato & Rice Soup	Rakusen	38.0	1.3	6.6	0.1	n/a
Tomato & Sausage Bontos	McVitie's	210	8.4	28.9	7.3	1.2
Tomato Chutney	Baxters	161 148	1.2 1.6	40.9 37.2	0.4 0.2	1.4 0.9
Tomato Juice		14.0	0.8	3.0	Tr	0.6
Tomato Juice Cocktail	Britvic	25.0	n/a	6.6	n/a	n/a
Tomato Ketchup		98.0	2.1	24.0	Tr	0.9
	Crosse & Blackwell	126	1.2	28.5	0.2	0.2

All amounts given per 100g/100ml unless otherwise stated

Product	Brand	Calories kcal	Protein (g)	Carbohydrate (g)	Fat (g)	Dietary Fibre (g)
	Heinz	104	1.0	24.9	Tr	1.3
	HP	111	1.2	28.3	Tr	n/a
healthy balance	Crosse & Blackwell	93.0	1.8	20.2	0.3	0.4
Tomato, Onion & Herb Pasta & Sauce	Batchelors	334	13.6	71.4	1.3	n/a
Tomato Pickle	Heinz Ploughman's	88.0	1.3	20.7	Tr	1.4
Tomato Puree		68.0	4.5	12.9	0.2	2.8
Tomato Relish	Branston	150	1.8	38.2	0.3	1.0
Tomato Rice Soup, condensed	Campbell's	93.0	1.6	17.1	2.0	0.4
Tomato Sauce		89.0	2.2	8.6	5.5	1.4
Tomato Sauce Crisps, per pack	Golden Wonder	153	2.0	12.2	10.6	n/a
Tomato Sauce Ringos, per pack	Golden Wonder	83.0	1.5	13.4	2.9	n/a
Tomato Soup						

canned, low calorie	Heinz Weight Watchers	25.0	0.6	4.5	0.5	0.7
condensed	Campbell's					
	Granny's Soup	56.0	1.1	10.9	0.9	0.7
dried, as sold		321	6.6	65.0	5.6	N
dried, as served		31.0	0.6	6.3	0.5	N
Tomato with Mushrooms & Herbs Pasta Sauce	Buitoni	96.0	1.8	19.8	0.8	0.8
Tomatoes, raw		17.0	0.7	3.1	0.3	1.0
fried in oil		91.0	0.7	5.0	7.7	1.3
grilled		49.0	2.0	8.9	0.9	2.9
canned		16.0	1.0	3.0	0.1	0.7
cherry, raw		18.0	0.8	3.0	0.4	1.0
Tongue, canned		213	16.0	nil	16.5	nil
Tooty Frooties	Rowntree Mackintosh	391	0.3	95.3	3.6	n/a
Top Cream Toffees, each	Trebor Bassett	36.0	n/a	5.3	1.6	n/a
Topic	Mars	483	7.4	56.7	26.7	n/a
Toppas	Kellogg's	360	9.0	74.0	2.0	8.0

All amounts given per 100g/100ml unless otherwise stated

Product	Brand	Calories kcal	Protein (g)	Carbo-hydrate (g)	Fat (g)	Dietary Fibre (g)
Tortellini Pot Meal	Boots Shapers	68.0	2.9	9.0	2.5	n/a
Tortelloni 5 Cheese	Dolmio	206	8.3	27.8	7.7	n/a
Tortelloni Italian Ham	Dolmio	184	8.6	25.9	5.8	n/a
Tortelloni Verona	Dolmio Ready Meals	145	4.5	12.9	8.7	n/a
Tortilla Chips		459	7.6	60.1	22.6	4.9
Toscano Salad Dressing	Napolina	587	1.4	3.4	62.6	n/a
Tostada Shells	Old El Paso	473	n/a	n/a	n/a	n/a
Totem Pole Mivvi, each	Lyons Maid	336	0.2	20.7	Tr	n/a
Tots (Rowntree Mackintosh): see flavours						
Tracker, choc chip roast nut	Mars Mars	490 503	9.1 10.0	56.3 52.8	26.9 29.4	n/a n/a
Traditional Beef Stewpot	Mr Brain's	124	4.9	12.3	6.5	n/a
Traditional Chocolate Sponge Mix, made up, per serving	Homepride Perfect	97.0	2.5	17.0	2.0	n/a
Traditional Crunchy Original						

Toasted Oats Cereal						
with bran & apple	Mornflake	380	11.0	52.0	12.0	14.0
with honey, almonds & raisins	Mornflake	390	12.0	60.0	11.5	14.0
with oat bran & nuts	Mornflake	361	10.5	60.0	12.0	12.0
Traditional Golden Pouring Syrup	Lyle's	284	Tr	76.0	nil	nil
Traditional Malt Bakes	McVitie's	502	5.9	67.0	22.9	1.8
Traditional Matzos	Rakusen	333	9.5	80.0	1.0	3.0
Traditional Morning Coffee Biscuits	Crawfords	466	6.9	75.4	14.5	2.3
Traditional Nice Biscuits	Crawfords	494	5.7	70.2	20.7	2.3
Traditional Ragu	Brooke Bond	79.0	1.9	12.1	2.8	n/a
Traditional Shortcake Biscuits	Crawfords	514	5.8	66.1	24.6	2.0
Traditional Sponge Mix, made up, per serving	Homepride Perfect	97.0	2.0	19.0	1.5	n/a
Traditional Tomato & Herbs Pasta Sauce	Buitoni	105	1.8	21.7	0.9	0.5

All amounts given per 100g/100ml unless otherwise stated

Product	Brand	Calories kcal	Protein (g)	Carbohydrate (g)	Fat (g)	Dietary Fibre (g)
Traditional Wholemeal Bread	Allinson	217	10.3	38.4	2.5	6.5
Trail Mix		432	9.1	37.2	28.5	4.3
Treacle, black		257	1.2	67.2	nil	nil
Treacle Sponge Pudding	Heinz	301	2.2	51.4	0.7	0.3
Treacle Tart		368	3.7	60.4	14.1	1.1
Treacle Tarts	Lyons	397	4.2	67.4	14.1	1.4
Treasure Crunch	Mornflake	400	12.2	60.0	13.0	14.0
Trebor Mints, each	Trebor Bassett	6.0	n/a	1.5	Tr	n/a
Trifle		160	3.6	22.3	6.3	0.5
with fresh cream		166	2.4	19.5	9.2	0.5
Trifle: see also flavours						
Trifle Mix, made up per serving, all flavours	Bird's	206	4.5	33.3	7.1	n/a
Trifle Sponge	Lyons	314	4.9	74.3	1.8	1.1
Trio Biscuits	Jacob's	529	5.0	59.8	31.6	0.5
Trio Choc Biscuits	Jacob's	518	5.5	59.7	30.3	0.5

Triple Choc Mivvi, each	Lyons Maid	208	1.9	15.5	15.8	n/a
Tripe, dressed *dressed, stewed*		60.0 / 100	9.4 / 14.8	nil / nil	2.5 / 4.5	nil / nil
Triple X Mints	Rowntree Mackintosh	371	0.6	98.3	nil	n/a
Tropical Drink, Fruit Burst	Del Monte	45.0	0.2	11.1	Tr	n/a
Tropical Fruit Cocktail	Del Monte	62.0	0.4	15.9	0.1	n/a
Tropical Fruit Drink	Boots Shapers	0.47	Tr	Tr	nil	nil
Tropical Fruit Solar	McVitie's	456	6.1	56.5	22.9	1.8
Tropical Juice Bar Mivvi, each	Lyons Maid	37.0	Tr	9.9	Tr	n/a
Tropical Mix	Ross	64.0	2.5	9.5	2.8	2.4
Tropical Prawns cooked & peeled in brine	Lyons / Lyons	53.0 / 71.0	12.0 / 14.3	nil / 2.0	0.6 / 0.7	n/a / n/a
Tropical Squash ready to drink	St Clements	42.8	0.1	11.5	Tr	n/a

All amounts given per 100g/100ml unless otherwise stated

Product	Brand	Calories kcal	Protein (g)	Carbo-hydrate (g)	Fat (g)	Dietary Fibre (g)
undiluted	St Clements	186	0.3	44.4	0.2	n/a
Tropical Yogurt Drink	Ski Cool	72.0	3.2	15.0	0.3	n/a
Trout, brown, steamed, flesh only		135	23.5	nil	4.5	nil
Tuc Biscuits	McVitie's	530	7.1	60.8	28.1	2.1
Tuc Savoury Sandwich Biscuits	McVitie's	571	8.0	49.5	37.5	1.5
Tuna						
canned in oil, drained		189	27.1	nil	9.0	nil
canned in brine, drained		99.0	23.5	nil	0.6	nil
Tuna & Mayonnaise Paste	Shippams	254	n/a	n/a	n/a	n/a
Tuna & Pasta Bake	Boots Shapers	82.0	6.1	6.7	3.6	1.1
Tuna & Pasta Pot Meal	Boots Shapers	111	7.8	10.0	4.7	n/a
Tuna & Pasta Salad	Boots	207	6.2	15.0	14.0	0.6
Tuna Canelloni	Heinz Weight Watchers	99.0	8.0	9.3	3.3	0.4
Tuna Crumble	Ross Recipe Meal	191	7.6	14.4	11.7	0.6

Tuna in Mayonnaise Sandwich Maker	Shippams	178	n/a	n/a	n/a	n/a	n/a
Tunes	Mars	368	nil	98.1	nil	nil	nil
Turkey, roast							
meat only		140	28.8	nil	2.7	nil	
meat & skin		171	28.0	nil	6.5	nil	
light meat		132	29.8	nil	1.4	nil	
dark meat		148	27.8	nil	4.1	nil	
Turkey & Ham Pie	Fray Bentos	169	9.6	16.2	7.8	n/a	
Turkey Roll, stuffed, canned	Tyne Brand	144	11.7	7.8	7.6	n/a	
Turkish Delight, without nuts	Cadbury	295	0.6	77.9	nil	nil	
per bar		180	1.0	37.5	4.1	n/a	
Turnip, boiled		12.0	0.6	2.0	0.2	1.9	
Turtles Bolognese	HP	95.0	4.1	12.7	3.1	0.7	
Tuscan Bean Soup	Rakusen	26.0	1.6	3.9	0.4	n/a	
Tutti Frutti Dairy Ice Cream	Lyons Maid Napoli	114	2.9	15.6	5.3	n/a	
Tutti Frutti Soya Ice Cream	Granose	96.0	1.2	14.4	3.4	n/a	

All amounts given per 100g/100ml unless otherwise stated

Product	Brand	Calories kcal	Protein (g)	Carbo-hydrate (g)	Fat (g)	Dietary Fibre (g)
Twiglets, large/small	Peek Frean	389	11.8	60.2	12.9	9.1
Twirl, per finger	Cadbury	115	1.9	12.5	6.6	n/a
Twix	Mars	479	5.8	63.5	24.2	n/a
Tzatziki		66.0	3.7	2.0	4.9	0.2

Umbongo Fruit Drink	Libby	43.0	Tr	10.7	Tr	Tr
apple	Libby	44.0	Tr	10.9	Tr	Tr
orange	Libby	42.0	Tr	10.3	Tr	Tr

Uncle Ben's Stir Fry Range: *see flavours*

United Biscuits

golden crunch	McVitie's	499	5.9	64.7	23.4	1.5
mint	McVitie's	499	5.8	67.0	23.1	1.5
orange	McVitie's	498	5.8	64.6	23.3	1.5

V8 Juice	Campbell's	20.0	0.8	4.0	0.1	nil
Vanilla & Strawberry Fromage Frais Split	Gold Ski	130	5.5	16.3	5.2	n/a
Vanilla Blancmange, as sold	Brown & Polson	328	0.4	86.9	0.1	n/a
Vanilla Dessert with a Caramel Sauce	Chamboury	108	3.3	22.8	0.8	Tr
Vanilla Ice Cream	Delight Wall's Blue	157	3.8	24.0	5.8	n/a

All amounts given per 100g/100ml unless otherwise stated

Product	Brand	Calories kcal	Protein (g)	Carbo-hydrate (g)	Fat (g)	Dietary Fibre (g)
cream of Cornish,	Ribbon	85.0	1.5	11.0	4.0	n/a
cream of Cornish,	Wall's	90.0	2.0	12.0	4.5	n/a
low fat	Wall's	80.0	2.0	12.0	3.0	n/a
reduced calorie	Heinz Weight Watchers	69.0	1.6	7.5	3.0	nil
soft scoop	Wall's Blue Ribbon	85.0	1.5	11.0	4.0	n/a
Vanilla Soya Ice Cream	Granose	89.0	1.2	12.5	3.4	n/a
Vanilla Yogurt, French style	St Ivel Shape	40.0	4.8	5.3	0.1	n/a
Veal						
cutlet, fried in oil		215	31.4	4.4	8.1	0.1
fillet, roast		230	31.6	nil	11.5	nil
Veal & Mushroom Pasta Sauce, dry, as sold	Buitoni	361	12.1	50.4	12.3	1.5
Vegelinks	Granose	167	20.1	11.7	4.7	1.5
Vegetable & Pasta Gratin	Findus Lean Cuisine	95.0	4.0	13.8	2.6	1.5

Vegetable Au Gratin	Granose	100	3.0	15.0	3.0	n/a
	Heinz Weight Watchers	73.0	3.2	8.9	2.7	1.2
Vegetable Bake	Ross Ready Meal	87.0	3.5	10.8	3.9	1.3
Vegetable Burgers, each	Birds Eye	80.0	6.5	5.0	4.0	n/a
Vegetable Casserole, canned	Campbell's	60.0	2.5	12.1	0.2	2.1
Vegetable Chilli	Heinz Weight Watchers	63.0	3.1	10.9	0.8	3.4
Vegetable Chilli Snack Pot	Boots Shapers	84.0	5.0	17.0	1.8	2.6
Vegetable Cubes	Knorr	315	11.6	22.8	20.3	1.8
Vegetable Curry canned with rice	Tyne Brand	57.0	2.0	9.6	1.4	n/a
	Heinz Weight Watchers	91.0	1.5	17.6	1.6	1.3
Vegetable Enchilladas	Findus Lean Cuisine	71.0	2.7	10.0	2.0	1.1
Vegetable Feasts, each	Birds Eye	427	2.0	13.0	5.0	n/a

All amounts given per 100g/100ml unless otherwise stated

Product	Brand	Calories kcal	Protein (g)	Carbo-hydrate (g)	Fat (g)	Dietary Fibre (g)
Vegetable Fingers, crispy, each	Birds Eye	45.0	1.0	5.0	2.5	n/a
Vegetable Ghee	Sharwood	897	Tr	Tr	99.7	n/a
Vegetable Gratin	Boots Shapers	111	6.1	13.0	4.2	2.0
Vegetable Gravy Granules, as sold	Brooke Bond	297	8.8	57.4	5.2	n/a
Vegetable Grills, original, each	Birds Eye	130	7.5	12.0	6.0	n/a
Vegetable Hotpot	Heinz Weight Watchers	66.0	2.8	8.9	2.1	1.5
Vegetable Korma Soup	Baxters	43.0	1.5	8.3	0.7	1.4
Vegetable Lasagne	Batchelors Microchef Meal	92.0	4.4	13.8	2.7	n/a
	Ross Ready Meal	110	5.3	12.6	4.7	0.9
per pack	Birds Eye Healthy Options	300	23.0	33.0	9.5	n/a
reduced calorie	Heinz Weight Watchers	69.0	3.9	9.7	1.6	0.7

Vegetable Margarine	Granose	750	0.1	0.1	83.0	n/a
Vegetable Moussaka	Heinz Weight Watchers	53.0	2.8	7.2	1.4	1.1
Vegetable Oil	Granose	899	Tr	nil	99.9	nil
Vegetable Pate	Granose	295	8.7	4.3	27.2	4.0
Vegetable Pie	Ross	266	6.1	27.8	15.8	3.0
Vegetable Pizza	McVitie's	162	7.0	25.2	4.6	2.1
Vegetable Quarter Pounders, original, each	Birds Eye	190	5.5	18.0	11.0	n/a
Vegetable Ravioli	Crosse & Blackwell	63.0	1.8	13.0	0.4	0.1
Vegetable Rice Choice, as sold	Crosse & Blackwell	363	8.4	74.2	3.6	4.0
Vegetable Risotto	Findus Lean Cuisine	94.0	2.9	14.9	2.5	1.5
Vegetable Salad	Eden Vale	124	1.4	8.0	9.8	n/a
	Heinz	155	1.7	13.2	10.6	1.6

All amounts given per 100g/100ml unless otherwise stated

Product	Brand	Calories kcal	Protein (g)	Carbohydrate (g)	Fat (g)	Dietary Fibre (g)
Vegetable Samosas: see Samosas						
Vegetable Soup, canned, ready to serve						
condensed	Campbell's	37.0	1.5	6.7	0.7	1.5
low calorie	Heinz Weight Watchers	59.0	1.6	12.5	0.3	1.5
		23.0	0.9	4.5	0.2	0.8
Vegetables Cantonese	Del Monte	74.0	1.3	11.7	2.5	n/a
Vegetables Caribbean	Del Monte	71.0	3.5	8.8	2.5	n/a
Vegetables in Chilli Stir Fry	Sharwood	63.0	1.2	10.9	1.7	1.4
Vegetables in Sweet & Sour Stir Fry	Sharwood	116	0.6	27.7	0.6	1.1
Vegetables Mexican	Del Monte	116	5.6	14.3	4.0	n/a
Vegetables South Sea Island	Del Monte	86.0	1.9	12.0	3.4	n/a
Vegetarian Cheddar	St Ivel	412	25.5	0.1	34.4	n/a
Vegetarian Cheeseburger	Granose	200	13.0	22.0	6.9	8.2
Vegetarian Double Gloucester	St Ivel	405	24.6	0.1	34.4	n/a
Vegetarian Mincemeat	Applefords	257	0.7	61.2	2.7	n/a

Vegetarian Party Links	Granose	346	7.9	3.8	33.2	n/a
Vegetarian Red Leicester	St Ivel	401	24.3	0.1	33.7	n/a
Vegetarian Sausages	Granose	190	6.7	12.0	13.0	4.5
Vegetarian Spicy Links	Granose	346	7.9	3.8	33.2	n/a
Venison, roast, meat only	Granose	198	35.0	nil	6.4	nil
Vermouth						
dry		118	0.1	5.5	nil	nil
sweet		151	Tr	15.9	nil	nil
Very Low Fat Spread (see also brands)		273	8.3	3.6	25.0	nil
Vessen Pate: see flavours						
Vesta Meals (Batchelors): see flavours						
Vichyssoise	Crosse & Blackwell	54.0	1.2	5.9	2.8	0.3
Victoria Sponge Mix, as sold	Homepride Classic	318	5.0	48.0	11.5	n/a
Viennese Whirls	Lyons	504	3.7	58.6	29.9	1.4
Viennetta Ice Cream (see also flavours)						

All amounts given per 100g/100ml unless otherwise stated

Product	Brand	Calories kcal	Protein (g)	Carbohydrate (g)	Fat (g)	Dietary Fibre (g)
individual	Wall's	150	2.0	14.0	10.0	n/a
original	Wall's	130	2.0	14.0	8.0	n/a
Vinaigrette Dressing, fat free	Kraft	40.0	Tr	10.0	Tr	n/a
Vindaloo Classic Curry Sauce	Homepride	55.0	1.9	8.7	n/a	n/a
Vindaloo Curry Paste	Sharwood	366	5.2	5.7	35.8	6.7
Vindaloo Curry Sauce, canned	Sharwood	88.0	2.2	6.0	6.2	1.6
Vindaloo Curry Sauce Mix, as sold	Sharwood	241	10.2	29.4	8.7	14.4
Vindaloo Hot Vegetable Curry	Holland & Barrett	82.0	2.1	11.5	3.5	0.9
Vintage Cider: see Cider						
Vintage Orange Marmalade	Baxters	200	Tr	53.0	Tr	0.8
Vitbe Bread, etc (Allied Bakeries): see flavours						

W

					N
Wafer Biscuits, filled		535	4.7	66.0	29.9
Wafer Cream	Tunnock's	513	6.6	63.2	28.0	n/a
Waffles: see Potato Waffles					
Waistline Dressings (Crosse & Blackwell): see flavours					
Walnut Cookies	Boots	506	6.0	59.0	29.0	2.8
Walnut Halves	Whitworths	525	10.6	5.0	51.5	5.2
Walnut Whip, milk chocolate vanilla flavour	Rowntree Mackintosh	488	5.7	63.7	25.1	n/a
Walnuts		688	14.7	3.3	68.5	3.5
Water Biscuits high bake	Jacob's	387	9.8	74.6	7.5	3.5

All amounts given per 100g/100ml unless otherwise stated

Product	Brand	Calories kcal	Protein (g)	Carbohydrate (g)	Fat (g)	Dietary Fibre (g)
rich	Jacob's	411	10.0	69.0	12.35	3.4
Water Chestnuts, canned		31.0	0.9	7.4	Tr	N
Watermelon: see Melon						
Weetabix	Weetabix	346	11.9	68.4	2.7	9.7
Weetaflakes	Weetabix	354	10.0	72.7	2.6	8.6
Weetos	Weetabix	388	6.2	80.5	4.6	4.6
Weight Watchers Products (Heinz): *see flavours*						
Wensleydale Cheese		377	23.3	0.1	31.5	nil
West Country Beef Layer Bake	Mr Brain's	149	6.2	9.9	9.7	n/a
West Country Chicken Hotpot	Mr Brain's	82.0	6.5	10.4	1.9	n/a
West Country Draught Cider	HP Bulmer	34.0	n/a	n/a	n/a	n/a
West Country Lamb Hotpot	Mr Brain's	115	6.6	9.9	5.8	n/a
West Country Sausage Casserole	Mr Brain's	142	3.7	12.0	9.2	n/a
West India Treacle	Fowler's	257	1.0	64.0	nil	nil

Wheat Flour: see Flour, wheat

Wheaten Matzos	Rakusen	340	9.9	78.0	1.0	5.0
Wheatgerm	Boots	302	26.7	44.7	9.2	15.6
	Jordans	379	27.0	50.0	9.3	2.7
natural		337	26.0	49.0	8.0	12.0
Wheatgerm Bread: see Bread						
Wheatgerm Oil		899	Tr	nil	99.9	nil
Wheatgrain Bread Mix, as sold	Homepride	264	11.0	50.0	2.0	n/a
Whelks, boiled, weighed with shells		14.0	2.8	Tr	0.3	nil
Whisky		224	nil	Tr	nil	nil
White Bread: see Bread & also flavours						
White Bread Mix, as sold	Homepride	263	10.0	48.0	3.0	n/a
White Cap Cooking Fat	Van Den Berghs	900	nil	nil	100	n/a
White Choc Chip Harvest Chewy Bar, each	Quaker	107	1.5	16.2	4.0	0.6
White Chocolate		529	8.0	58.3	30.9	nil
diabetic	Boots	485	9.8	51.0	34.0	0.2

All amounts given per 100g/100ml unless otherwise stated

Product	Brand	Calories kcal	Protein (g)	Carbo-hydrate (g)	Fat (g)	Dietary Fibre (g)
White Chocolate Coated Lemon Lunchbar	Boots Shapers	448	7.6	64.0	18.0	n/a
White Chocolate Ice cream	Wall's Carte D'Or	160	2.0	14.0	12.0	n/a
White Corn	Green Giant	64.0	n/a	n/a	0.7	n/a
White Pepper: see Pepper						
White Pudding		450	7.0	36.3	31.8	N
White Rice: see Rice						
White Rolls: see Bread Rolls						
White Sauce						
savoury, made with whole milk		150	4.1	10.9	7.8	0.2
savoury, made with semi-skimmed milk		128	4.2	11.1	10.3	0.2
sweet, made with whole milk		170	3.8	18.6	9.5	0.2
sweet, made with semi-skimmed milk		150	3.9	18.8	7.2	0.2
White Stilton Cheese: see Stilton						
White Wine, dry		66.0	0.1	0.6	nil	nil
medium		75.0	0.1	3.4	nil	nil
sparkling		76.0	0.2	5.9	nil	nil

sweet		94.0	0.2	5.9	nil	nil
White Wine Casserole Recipe Sauce	Knorr	81.0	1.8	7.8	4.9	n/a
White Wine Cook-In-Sauce						
can	Homepride	57.0	0.6	7.2	n/a	n/a
jar	Homepride	68.0	1.0	9.6	n/a	n/a
Whitebait, fried		525	19.5	5.3	47.5	0.2
	Young's	118	16.0	nil	5.3	n/a
Golden	Young's	283	12.1	16.0	19.2	0.7
Whiting, steamed, flesh only		92.0	20.9	nil	0.9	nil
in crumbs, fried		191	18.1	7.0	10.3	0.3
Whole Milk: see Milk						
Whole Soups (Heinz): see flavours						
Wholegrain Mustard	Colman's	164	8.5	n/a	10.0	n/a
Wholegrain Rice						
	Uncle Ben's	114	2.8	24.1	0.8	n/a
3 minute, canned	Uncle Ben's	103	2.6	22.0	1.0	n/a
frozen	Uncle Ben's	147	3.7	30.9	1.8	n/a
Whole Rye Crispbread	Boots Shapers	367	9.5	8.3	2.0	2.9

All amounts given per 100g/100ml unless otherwise stated

Product	Brand	Calories kcal	Protein (g)	Carbohydrate (g)	Fat (g)	Dietary Fibre (g)
Wholegrain Fruit Muesli	Granose	392	8.1	74.8	6.1	n/a
Wholegrain Mustard: see Mustard						
Wholemeal Baps	Hovis	215	10.7	34.5	3.2	5.0
Wholemeal/Wholewheat Bread: see Bread						
Wholemeal Crackers		413	10.1	72.1	11.3	4.4
Wholemeal Flour, see Flour, wholemeal						
Wholemeal Hot Cross Buns	Hovis	258	9.8	42.6	6.7	4.4
Wholemeal Malt Loaf	Allinson	259	10.6	48.2	2.6	6.8
Wholemeal Muffins, each	Allinson	143	7.3	25.1	1.6	4.5
Wholemeal Pasta & Smoked Ham Salad, per pack	Boots	263	n/a	n/a	n/a	n/a
Wholemeal Pastry: see Pastry						
Wholemeal Pitta, each	International Harvest	157	7.7	28.6	1.2	4.9
mini, each	International Harvest	68.0	3.4	12.5	0.5	2.1

Wholemeal Rolls, each	Allinson	116	5.4	17.9	2.2	2.7
Wholemeal Scones: see Scones						
Wholemeal Scotch Rolls	Hovis	230	11.3	37.6	3.2	5.3
Wholenut Chocolate	Cadbury	560	9.5	48.2	37.9	n/a
Wholewheat Macaroni: see Macaroni						
Wholewheat Noodles	Sharwood	334	13.1	68.4	2.8	10.1
Wholewheat Ravioli: see Ravioli						
Wholewheat Spaghetti: see Spaghetti						
Wild Strawberry Yogurt	Alpine Ski	90.0	5.0	17.1	0.7	n/a
Willow Spread	Dairy Crest	709	0.7	1.0	78.0	nil
Wine: see flavours						
Wine Gums	Trebor Bassett	326	4.0	78.7	Tr	nil
Winkles, boiled, weighed with shells		14.0	2.9	Tr	0.3	nil
Winner Choc Bar, each	Wall's	203	3.3	19.5	13.0	n/a
Winter Vegetable Soup	Heinz	47.0	2.8	8.7	0.1	2.1
Wispa, per standard bar	Cadbury	210	2.9	20.7	13.6	n/a

All amounts given per 100g/100ml unless otherwise stated

Product	Brand	Calories kcal	Protein (g)	Carbo-hydrate (g)	Fat (g)	Dietary Fibre (g)
Woodpecker Cider						
bottles/can	HP Bulmer	29.0	n/a	n/a	n/a	n/a
draught	HP Bulmer	35.0	n/a	n/a	n/a	n/a
dry	HP Bulmer	30.0	n/a	n/a	n/a	n/a
Woppa Chews, each	Trebor Bassett	18.0	Tr	3.8	0.2	n/a
Worcester Ketchup	Lea & Perrins	69.0	0.3	14.6	1.0	n/a
Worcestershire Sauce	Lea & Perrins	115	1.5	25.6	0.6	n/a

Product	Brand	Calories kcal	Protein (g)	Carbo-hydrate (g)	Fat (g)	Dietary Fibre (g)
Yam, raw		114	1.5	28.2	0.3	1.3
boiled		133	1.7	33.0	0.3	1.4
Yeast, bakers, compressed		53.0	11.4	1.1	0.4	N

						N
dried		169	35.6	3.5	1.5	
Yellow Bean Stir Fry Sauce	Sharwood	129	0.3	28.9	1.7	1.5
Yellow Split Peas, boiled	Whitworths	118	8.3	21.9	0.3	5.1
Yes Cakes, chocolate	Rowntree Mackintosh	442	6.6	50.0	25.4	n/a
caramel	Rowntree Mackintosh	442	6.3	50.0	25.5	n/a
Yogonaise	Delight	42.0	0.2	2.0	3.8	Tr
Yogurt (see also flavours)						
Greek style, cows		115	6.4	2.0	9.1	nil
Greek style, sheep		106	4.4	5.6	7.5	nil
low calorie		41.0	4.3	6.0	0.2	N
low fat, plain		56.0	5.1	7.5	0.8	N
low fat, flavoured		90.0	3.8	17.9	0.9	N
low fat, fruit		90.0	4.1	17.9	0.7	N
soya		72.0	5.0	3.9	4.2	N
whole milk, plain		79.0	5.7	7.8	3.0	N
whole milk, fruit		105	5.1	15.7	2.8	N
Yogurt & Cucumber Dip	Burgess	498	3.9	13.3	47.0	Tr

All amounts given per 100g/100ml unless otherwise stated

Product	Brand	Calories kcal	Protein (g)	Carbo-hydrate (g)	Fat (g)	Dietary Fibre (g)
Yogurt & Cucumber Dressing	Burgess	325	2.1	17.1	27.1	0.1
Yogurt, French style, all varieties	Eden Vale	101	3.8	15.1	3.2	n/a
Yogurt & Chive Dressing	Heinz All Seasons	295	1.5	13.9	25.9	nil
Yorkie (Rowntree Mackintosh): *see flavours*						
Young Broad Beans, 1oz/28g	Birds Eye	17.0	2.0	2.0	Tr	n/a
Young Sweetcorn, 1oz/28g	Birds Eye	30.0	1.0	6.0	0.5	n/a
Yorkshire Pudding		208	6.6	24.7	9.9	0.9
Yorkshire Pudding & Pancake Mix, as sold	Whitworths	348	12.6	76.6	1.1	nil
YoYo (McVitie's): *see flavours*						
Yum Yums	Sunblest	455	5.8	45.5	27.8	1.0

Z

Zabaglione Classic Dessert	Chambourcy	205	3.7	22.0	11.0	0.2
Zoom, each	Lyons Maid	47.0	0.3	10.0	0.5	n/a
Zucchini: *see Courgettes*						
Zucchini Lasagne	Findus Lean Cuisine	64.0	5.0	7.9	1.4	1.6

All amounts given per 100g/100ml unless otherwise stated

COLLINS GEM

Other Gem titles that may interest you include:

Gem Healthy Eating and Nutrition
A compact guide to the nutritional values of
everyday foodstuffs and drinks **£2.99**

Gem Food Additives
An invaluable directory of over 1300 terms relating
to food additives **£2.99**

Gem Food for Freezing
Describes food suitable for freezing, food
preparation techniques, and freezing and
thawing methods **£2.99**

Gem Food for Microwaving
Contains everything you need to know about
microwaving food at home **£2.99**

Gem Vegetarian Food
Describes over 600 vegetarian foodstuffs with
information on preparation and uses **£2.99**

Gem Herbs for Cooking and Health
Details how to grow and use the range of herbs that
have traditionally been used in cooking and
medicine **£3.50**

COLLINS GEM

Bestselling Collins Gem titles include:

Gem English Dictionary (£3.50)
Gem Calorie Counter (£2.99)
Gem Thesaurus (£2.99)
Gem French Dictionary (£3.50)
Gem German Dictionary (£3.50)
Gem Basic Facts Mathematics (£2.99)
Gem Birds (£3.50)
Gem Babies' Names (£3.50)
Gem Card Games (£3.50)
Gem Atlas of the World (£3.50)

All Collins Gems are available from your local bookseller or can be ordered direct from the publishers.

In the UK, contact Mail Order, Dept 2M, HarperCollins Publishers, Westerhill Rd, Bishopbriggs, Glasgow, G64 2QT, listing the titles required and enclosing a cheque or p.o. for the value of the books plus £1.00 for the first title and 25p for each additional title to cover p&p. Access and Visa cardholders can order on 041-772 2281 (24 hr).

In Australia, contact Customer Services, HarperCollins Distribution, Yarrawa Rd, Moss Vale 2577 (tel. [048] 68 0300). **In New Zealand**, contact Customer Services, HarperCollins Publishers, 31 View Rd, Glenfield, Auckland 10 (tel. [09] 444 3740). **In Canada**, contact your local bookshop.

All prices quoted are correct at time of going to press.